ONE STEP:
How I Took One Step to Lose 600lbs.

DELUXE EDITION
Featuring Bonus "The One Step Method"

By: Justin Willoughby

© Justin Willoughby, 2017
http://onestepnation.com
http://justinwilloughby.com

All things are possible!

Table of Contents

Chapter 1: One Step (The Journey Begins) 5

Chapter 2: It's Time to Choose 14

Chapter 3 – The Journey 24

Chapter 4: THE SET BACKS 34

Chapter 5: I'm Alive Again 46

Chapter 6 – The Steps Towards Weight Loss 59

Chapter 7: ONE STEP NATION 72

Chapter 8: Your Only Hope 79

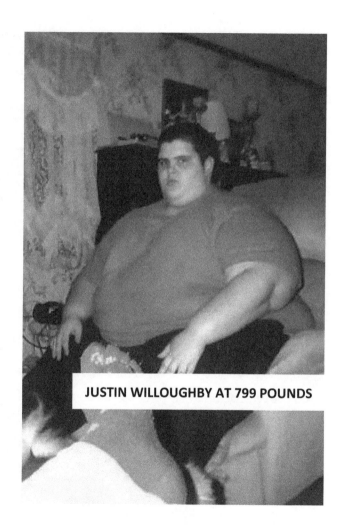
JUSTIN WILLOUGHBY AT 799 POUNDS

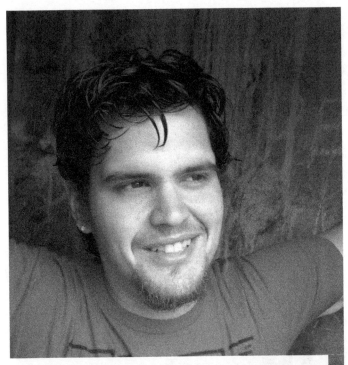
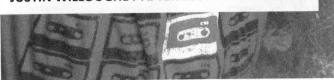
JUSTIN WILLOUGHBY AFTER LOSING 600 POUNDS

Chapter 1: One Step (The Journey Begins)

It was like a bad dream. One day my Mother informed me that it was time for a visit to my doctor. If I didn't see him soon, I would no longer be covered by the insurance company that we had. I couldn't go to a doctor, I thought ; I hadn't been out of my house trailer in over eight months. I wasn't even sure if I could walk, let alone go see a doctor. I was huge! There was no denying this. I had always struggled with a weight issue my whole life, however, I'd never been this large.

My Father helped me stand up in my bedroom. He walked me over to the hallway and he helped me down the cement stairway that led into my house trailer. I waddled about 30 feet to the 2002 Oldsmobile Intrigue. My Father opened the door and I set one leg in. I was so nervous, it had been so long since I'd sat in a vehicle. I laid down sideways in the back seat, and my Dad pushed my leg into the vehicle so I could fit better. He slammed the door quickly before my foot fell out of the current position that it was in. There I was, crushed like a sardine in the back seat, lying sideways on my way to the doctor's office. The doctor must have been expecting me because they were waiting for me with a wheelchair that was made for the morbidly obese. I sat in the wheelchair, but I couldn't fit through the door. I stood up, and walked a few feet down the hall, until I could sit in the wheelchair and fit through the hallway. My parents wheeled me into the doctor's office. I remember feeling so humiliated and out of place. This was something I wasn't happy about. I didn't want to face the issues that I was having. I didn't want a doctor telling me that I weighed too much, or that I had to lose weight. I mean, was I really that big? Did I really need to lose weight? I felt how large I was, but I didn't understand the urgency behind it. Why couldn't my parents and doctors just mind their own business? I wanted to live life my way. Nobody needed to tell me what to do. Everything was fine at home.

The doctor and nurse came out, and their facial expression said it all to me. I knew I was large, but how large was I? They checked my vitals and they seemed very concerned about me, due to my size. One nurse burst into tears. She couldn't believe what happened to me since she last saw me, which was roughly about 4 years prior to this. The doctor talked to my parents for what seemed like forever, and then they sent me home. As I left the doctor's office I remember asking my parents to stop and buy me some donuts and a fruit soft drink. It had been a while since I ate, so they picked up a dozen donuts and gave me the fruit soft drink. I remember demolishing four donuts as soon as I got home. It comforted me and made me forget about all the embarrassment I just went through at the doctor's office. We were unaffected by what had just happened at the doctor's office. I didn't let the surprised look from the doctor worry me. I still had an appetite.

Isn't denial funny like that? We appear to be blind to ourselves and to our problems and situations, and if someone calls us out on something, how dare they! The donuts sounded way too good to pass up. Nobody was going to tell me if it was right or wrong to eat them. My parents didn't seem to understand the urgency of my weight problem, as they allowed me to eat more junk, even after being told of concerns that the doctor had with me being so large. Later, when my parents were asked why they allowed me to eat so much that caused me to gain so much weight, they simply talked about how they felt bad denying my requests out of love. They thought that their son deserved to be happy. Little did they know, due to their ignorance and passivity, I was in a situation that very few people even dream about getting out of. I don't fault my parents for how large I became. I was the one who chose to eat the food. I allowed addiction to make me balloon up to an insane amount of weight. They were ignorant of the reality in front of them.

    As time went on, I began understanding that I wasn't happy with myself. I hated what I'd become, but I wasn't sure what I'd become. I didn't know how much I weighed. I didn't know how large I was, since I avoided mirrors as if they would kill me. Now don't get me wrong; I knew I needed to do something about my weight, but I didn't know what I needed to do for sure, or even where to start. I was lost and pretty much blind to the dangerous reality in front of me. You'd think my eyes would have been opened a long time ago, like when my clothes were getting tighter and new clothes had to be purchased. I even had to sleep sitting up, due to the bad anxiety attacks I was having, and due to the difficulty breathing from being so large. If I laid down to sleep, I couldn't breathe well. I woke up gasping for air. It was terrifying. I couldn't even use the bathroom by myself, and I didn't have a social life. I lost most of my friends from my inactivity and from sitting inside so often. I didn't want my friends to see me, as I was aware that I was a lot bigger than them. It made me feel self-conscious and inferior. The smaller my world became, the larger I became.

    I was in bad shape, but I didn't grasp it deeply enough to want to experience transformation. When was all this going to change? When could I be a normal teenager again? Am I going to be like this forever? Will I get married? All these questions ran through my head. I was always a bit optimistic, so I usually believed the best in every situation. I went on living life like normal, or at least trying to act like life was normal. I sat on my bed and messed around with my desktop computer that was next to my bed. I asked my brother to make me an abundance of food and bring it to me. I took advantage of my brother quite frequently. My brother is autistic. I used that to my advantage. He never fully grasped my situation. He just wanted to make his little brother happy. So, I sent him to make me food, to buy me food from the convenience store that was only a 30 second walk from my home, and even periodically tricked him into giving me a portion of his food.

    I thought life was going to continue as it was, but I thought wrong. The day after my doctor's appointment, I heard the phone ring and then, the sound of my Mom crying. She came walking into my bedroom, upset and sobbing. She informed me about the phone call she just received. It was from the doctor's office that I had just seen. They told my mother that I needed to get help and help had to happen very quickly. My life was in danger, according to this doctor. I quickly rejected my mom's proposal of the ambulance coming to get me the next day to take me to Pittsburgh, PA's Children's Hospital. She told me I had to go. I was persistent, though. I kept screaming, "no"! I wasn't going. She told me this was a serious thing and that I could die if I didn't get checked out. I reluctantly agreed, but I wasn't happy about it. Tears started rolling down my face. Why did things have to change? Why did people have to get involved in my personal life? I wasn't ready for this. I wasn't ready for change. Everything was going to be so different. I was mad, sad and frustrated. My mom was a good talker. She could get me out of negative situations. Why couldn't she get me out of this one, too? I didn't need a doctor to tell me that I had to lose weight. What did this mean for my family? What did this mean for me? I wasn't excited about what was to come. This was going to be another embarrassing moment that I would remember forever. When will this ever end?

    The next day came very quickly. It appeared to happen in the blink of an eye. I was dreading the hour of the ambulance crew's arrival. I remember hearing the knock on the door and my stomach sank. I knew what it was time for. The medical staff came rushing into my room and they began talking to me. They assured me that I was going to be fine, and that they needed to take me to Pittsburgh for some testing. I began to be fearful. I didn't want to be separated from my parents. I didn't want to leave my hometown of Bradford, Pennsylvania. I just wanted this nightmare to end. I wanted to wake up and find that this was just a dream. With medical staff supporting me, one on each side, I remember the view that was waiting for me outside like it was yesterday. There was an ambulance crew waiting for me along with a fire and rescue team. It reminded me of something you would watch on TV. This couldn't be happening to me. This was Discovery channel material. This happened to other people. Never in a million years had I imagined this was going to be me one day, but it was. They took me downstairs and brought me to a stretcher. I couldn't fit on the stretcher that they provided, so they put me on the medical gurney. I was on the ground looking up at the cloudy sky in the summer of 2003. A few of the crew members tried to lift me via the gurney into the ambulance, but they couldn't. A few more crew members came over and they tried together; finally, it took at least 8 crew members to lift me into the ambulance. I didn't know what to expect next. The journey to my new life had begun.

    The ambulance started moving and my parents followed behind them in their vehicle. The next hour was very uncomfortable. The gurney was not designed for someone of my weight, nor for someone to lay on for hours. I had to get off of the gurney, because I couldn't get comfortable. I developed a bed sore instantaneously. They took me to another hospital where they put me in a better fitting ambulance. After what seemed like an eternity, we finally arrived to Pittsburgh's Children's Hospital. They wheeled me into the Emergency Room and took my vitals. My oxygen level was 60%, and my resting heart rate was 133 beats per minute. They ran some tests on me and then sent me to my room where my parents were waiting for me, along with my brother and a few nurses.

    Tears filled my eyes and I began feeling insecure, hopeless and scared. How could I let myself get this big? Tears were streaming down my face and my parents tried to comfort me. It didn't work. I was still battling the ultimate reality in front of me. To make matters worse, my parents looked at me and asked me if I wanted to know how much I weighed. I was hesitant at first, but I needed to hear it. My mom looked over at my dad and began to tear up. My mom whispered my weight into my ear. She told me I weighed 799 pounds. I was in utter shock. Something like blinders fell off of my eyes and finally it all sunk in. I was 799 pounds at the age of 16. I was just a teenager. I couldn't believe it. How did this happen? I began to cry and then I became numb. It was an extremely difficult moment, as so many emotions were running rampant in my mind. I didn't know how to handle the news that I just received. I didn't know what would happen to me next. With all my emotions flooding at full intensity, I was lost for words. My parents helped me get comfortable and turned the TV on for me. They left for the night, promising they would come back first thing in the morning to visit me. They both gave me a huge hug and told me they loved me.

It was a restless night of sleep. Doctors come in and out to do blood work and blood pressure checks nearly all night long. Noises from other patients, and the Pittsburgh morning traffic filled my ears for most of the time I spent at that hospital. It was far from the most restful sleep, that's for sure. The doctors came first thing in the morning and explained my situation to me. I finally began grasping that I needed help in order to survive this situation that I had gotten myself into. They told me about the tests they were going to do to see if I was clear of heart disease, cancer, diabetes, high blood pressure, and so on. They informed me that I would be put on a low calorie, low fat diet. "Oh great," I thought, "cardboard and water. I can hardly wait." I was accustomed to flavor, so this was going to take some getting used to.

My parents came walking in after the doctors left the room and I began to feel a little more hopeful. They informed me that they were there for me, and were going to find the help I needed to get me through this. After plenty of poking and prodding, people coming and going, it was finally determined that I had no life-threatening disorders. They did put me on oxygen, due to my levels being so far from normal. I was relieved that there were no major issues, besides sleep apnea and low oxygen.

Another day went by and my parents left for the night. I couldn't wait for this hospital visit to be over. As I was lying in bed, I remember a janitor coming into my room. He told me that I was going to be okay and that I was going to make it. His words really encouraged me and built up my self-esteem. Finally, a little bit of hope. "Maybe I can beat this!" I thought. Maybe I could shed all of those unwanted pounds and get my life back. It sounded crazy, but I was bound and determined to do something about this, even if it meant I would die trying.

I needed to understand the reality of the situation that I was facing. This was life or death for me. Either I do something to change or my life would be over. The question was, "Where do I start? How do I start? Who will help me?" It literally felt as if I was living on a prayer.

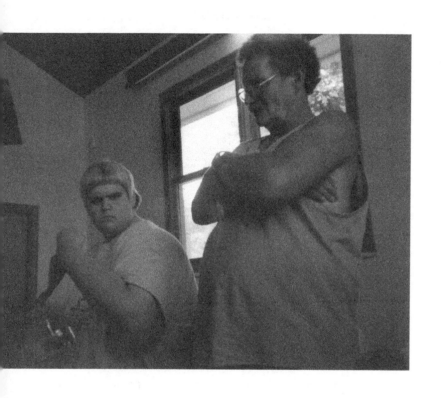

Chapter 2: It's Time to Choose

Choosing LIFE or DEATH became the next biggest decision of my life. If I continued down the road I was on, I was guaranteed to die. If I chose to do something about my train wreck of a life, I'd have a chance of living and maybe having a normal life. I had a blue Bible that I set on my hospital bed stand. I kept it with me as a type of good luck charm. I slept with this Bible, even taking it with me to my friend's house, keeping it in my pillow that I brought when I spent the night. I had it for a while. As I struggled with my dilemma, I remembered some words from my Bible. I recalled the story of Jesus and pondered what it meant for me. I had a choice to make. Obviously, I was wrecking my life by being enslaved to my unending appetite. I was on a downward spiral of destruction. The way I was living life certainly wasn't working for me. I was doing things all wrong. My view of life was skewed. I was destroying myself by living my own way. I felt hopeless. I was at the rock bottom of my life. Here I was, a 16-year-old teenager who didn't feel accepted by the culture, hated the way he looked, was unsure if he would ever get married and have children one day, and who was unsure if he'd live or die. I was completely broken and lost. I needed some intervention and a hope to hold onto.

I decided to give my life to Jesus. I know that sounds confusing to some people, but I had to place my life into the hands of Someone who I believe created life. I believed that with Jesus leading me, I would have an opportunity to have a new start at life and possibly lose weight and become a healthier person. This was a very important decision to make. The words I spoke weren't anything special. I wasn't a theologian nor was I a scholar in religion or faith. In fact, the words that I said, they were very basic.

You don't have to be a deep spiritually rooted person to call on Jesus. You just have to recognize that without Him, your life will not be life that is truly life. It's funny how we live as if we are truly alive, but when we surrender control so He can give us a new life, that's when we truly become alive. I thought I was alive before I trusted in Jesus. My life before coming to Him was a joke. Yet, He loved me just as I was, and gave me an opportunity to say yes to His approach to life. It was the best decision of my life.

I didn't notice extreme changes, at first. However, I did notice that my view of life and my situation became hopeful. A feeling of peace enveloped me. To be honest, I really didn't know if I was going to live or die. I felt as if I had gone too far to ever get back to normal. I completely understood that my life might not have a fairytale ending. I didn't want to die, but part of me figured that it was a realistic possibility. I had let myself go and abused the body that God had given me. I couldn't blame God for my life potentially being cut short. I could only blame myself. He gave me many opportunities to say no to food. I just didn't want to. The cravings were too strong. The flavors were too good. The feeling that food gave me was just too great to pass up. It's easy to blame God for circumstances that He didn't even put us in. He allows us to suffer the consequences of becoming enslaved to substances like food. He never intends to harm us, but He lets us see what happens when we go off on our own stubborn way. We were made to desire Him more than any substance. I just didn't realize that with my skewed view of life.

With my new-found faith, and the hope that it brought me, it was time to have a new outlook on life. When I was hospitalized, my attitude towards the doctors who ran tests was, "hurry up and get this over with, I want to go home." To my amazement, all my tests came back negative. I was a healthy young man in a 799-pound body. Fortunately, the only problems I had was low oxygen and sleep apnea, which were both weight related. It was such a blessing to not have developed heart disease or diabetes. Things began to look hopeful. I felt as if God's hand of blessing and protection was on my life. I adored how He didn't look at me like some fat freak who didn't matter. I didn't love myself. I regarded myself as ugly and insecure. Why would anyone but my family love me? My mindset was all wrong. I had a distorted view of love. Love to me was superficial and conditional. Thankfully, I began to understand that wasn't anything like God's love. He looked past my flaws and imperfections and saw His child who was lost and hurting. I found acceptance and meaning in my existence with Jesus. It changed my life. Just seeing the blessings that came with my trust in Him amazed me. I was able to witness the fingerprints of God all over my life. I could have chosen to ignore or and reject His signs. I could have been mad at God for allowing me to be in this situation. I could have rejected the opportunity to know Him deeper and more personally. My choices mattered.

After making up my mind to choose life, it was time for me to actually get to work and lose the unwanted weight. It was time to apply the diet and exercise program that the hospital staff had given me to recover. They put me on a diet that they told me to follow. I reluctantly gave in, and by doing so, I was on my way to shedding the unwanted weight that held me down and robbed me of an excellent and abundant life. I began to feel better quickly by choosing to apply their instructions and eat the way they wanted me to eat. I did miss the taste of flavorful foods, but I was looking forward to getting healthier and losing weight. The doctors had given me instructions to walk a few feet at a time, in order to start my recovery. Any type of activity was hard for me to do. It was difficult to move any part of my body. If I stood up, my back and legs cramped and developed spasms due to the immense stress of my weight. When I took steps, my heart rate escalated, causing me to have a panic attack. I had to choose to look past the negatives and look at those moments as moments of potential recovery and hope.

As hard as things were physically, the toughest battle was in my mind. I had to choose to stay positive and hopeful, even when my mind wanted to doubt and think negatively. I could no longer think as a defeated person. I had to think of myself as a person who was approaching this weight obstacle knowing that I would ultimately be victorious. A victor mindset helped me say, "yes" to staying faithful to my recovery plan. The great support I had from my parents and doctors helped keep my mind in check. I had to remember the promises of Jesus that He would never leave me nor forsake me. Mentally, I was becoming a new person. The old me would think negative thoughts that would wreck my self-esteem and self-image. I lived under a cloud of constant fear of dying. Fear interfered with my thought processes and caused me to limit my activities. Fear of dying kept me from living. However, since I put my trust in God, though the fear was still there, it was not as overwhelming. I was at the most peace in my life after coming to realize that I was powerless on my own.

Learning to gradually overcome fear was a huge step, given my mental health history. When I was 14 years old, I was diagnosed with anxiety and panic attack disorder. I didn't do anything active because I believed my heart would explode. My mind was always so full of anxiety and panic. Anxiety and panic attacks are what accelerated my weight gaining process. I remember waking up one night having to use the bathroom. I walked to the bathroom in the dead of night in a quiet home where everyone else was sleeping. As I walked back to bed after washing my hands, my heart started beating at a gradually faster pace. I began to feel overwhelmed and anxious. I began to hyperventilate and panic. Thoughts of death and hopelessness overwhelmed me. I ran to wake up my parents and frantically told them I was having a heart attack. I didn't know what else it could be. They rushed me to the emergency room where the nurses hooked me up to take my vitals, finding my heart rate was elevated and my blood pressure was high. After a few hours, everything went back to normal and I was discharged. The medical professionals couldn't figure out exactly what was wrong with me. The next day, I was sitting on my couch, watching TV and it happened again. I ran outside to get my parents and they rushed me to the emergency room once again. This time the medical professionals admitted me to the hospital to run some tests. Part of me was scared; the other part of me was glad, because I believed they would now figure out what was going on with me.

After three days of stress, as I had multiple tests and consultations with physicians, they concluded that I was experiencing anxiety attacks. My official diagnosis was anxiety and panic disorder. From that point on, fear became my new arch nemesis. Knowing my diagnosis didn't prevent me from being held captive to fear. Fear held me back from doing what my friends were doing. Things like going outside to play, going to a movie, going to a store and everything else a normal teenager does were impossible for me. I was prescribed anxiety medications that only numbed me but never fixed the problems that I was having. The medicine was like a Band-Aid over a gaping wound. Fear consumed me to the point where I took comfort only with food, using it to dismiss the thoughts of fear and panic. Eating numbed my emotions and took away all of my negative thoughts, temporarily. Food became my friend that helped me defeat fear. However, fear and food were both culprits that contributed to my insane amount of weight gain. Fear held me to a lifestyle of extremely limited activity because I was always assuming that if I moved, my heart would explode and I'd be a goner. Not feeling free to move meant that my body did not burn off the excess calories I was consuming. It was a nightmare that seemed like I would never wake up from. I was stuck in this insane rut that almost led to my demise.

    I was also haunted with questions such as, "What did I do to deserve having anxiety attacks?" I didn't have an answer. I was fearful of being left alone, due to the fear of potentially dying and nobody being around to help me or to comfort me in the process. Living a life of fear was no fun. Some nights, my dad slept next to me and rubbed my back to calm me down during my anxious moments. Every day was a mental struggle.

I went to see a psychologist and a psychiatrist, who both tried to help me. Now, I'm not a person that gives the devil the blame for everything that happens in life. However, since medication, physicians and other well- meaning people could not help me, I concluded that the source of my problems must be spiritual. I felt as if I was being held in bondage to fear and negative thinking. It stole my joy. It stole my will to live. It stole my personality. It stole my ability to be a normal person. Nothing that doctors could do provided any relief. I ended up in the ER countless times thinking that I was dying of a heart attack. I needed help beyond what anyone could offer.

I found the first peace in my life when I put my trust in Jesus. When I lined my thinking up to what He said about me, it melted away my anxiety. When I took my focus off Him, the anxiety returned. Before I found peace, I was on four different medications to help subside the anxious racing thoughts. I don't recommend doing this, but I finally decided enough was enough, and I quit all my medicines cold turkey. I was tired of being medicated due to something that held me in fear. I no longer wanted to be that person. Instead, I became a prayer warrior. I began believing what God said about me. I began having a new outlook. With bumps and bruises along the way, I ended up being SET FREE from anxiety attacks. What a tremendous blessing! I don't believe medicine is evil. I believe it's a tool to help us in our time of need. But for me, my anxiety was really a spiritual problem and so the solution was a spiritual answer. I am thankful that I chose that direction.

I am still not always anxiety free to this very day. I am still a normal guy and I get stressed and tensed. But now I am a person who doesn't allow a negative thought life to control me. I have to control it. Transformation starts with the renewing of our minds. Choices matter in all the situations that we find ourselves in. Will we choose the road that will give us the best results, even if it's hard? Or will we choose the easy road that will bring mediocre results, enslaved forever? I am happy that I chose the road that I did. By choosing to stay heavenly minded, I was able to get my life back from the clutches of negativity.

When was the last time you sat down and thought about your life? When was the last time you looked at your current health condition or spiritual condition? When was the last time you evaluated who you are? I believe evaluating our lives can lead us to transformation. Evaluating helps us see clearly where we are at, at this moment, and it helps us set our hopes and efforts towards a direction that will help us change for the better. If I continued to be blind to my condition when I was 799lbs, I would surely have continued down the path of destruction and most likely would not even be here to encourage you and inspire you to become a better version of yourself.

If you are reading this book, and you feel as if you are stuck in a rut and you feel hopeless, understand that you have to choose to perceive your situation in a different manner. You have to choose to change your approach to how you currently view your life. If you see that your situation is one that needs change, and you just sit and dwell on your current circumstance, you'll more than likely stay in that rut. Change requires you to get your focus off of hopelessness and focus on hopefulness. Don't allow your circumstances of addiction, lack of self-control, insecurities, anxiety, habits, depression, relationships, negative spirituality or anything else to rule your emotions or define your self-worth. Don't let the negative capture you and enslave you in a cage of hopelessness. You are worth more than what you believe you are worth. You can lose weight. You can overcome that addiction. You can see victory. You can restore broken relationships. You can be loved by God. You are an overcomer. It all comes down to choice. Do you believe this? Will you choose this mindset? If you do, you have to believe it in your heart and act as if you do. Setbacks will come, but should never influence you to quit; use setbacks to fall forward. We keep fighting like a fighter in the ring. One punch doesn't keep us down. We fight until we have nothing left, or until we take our last breath.

Choose life! Choose hope! Choose to cooperate with a Heavenly Father that loves you! Choose to dismiss the negative thoughts. Choose to embrace the change you need to become the best version of yourself. This is how I lost 600lbs. Some of us have 600lbs pounds of baggage to lose, not just physical weight. It's time to take those steps necessary to make that happen. I believe in you! That's why I felt compelled to write this book. CHOOSE WISELY!

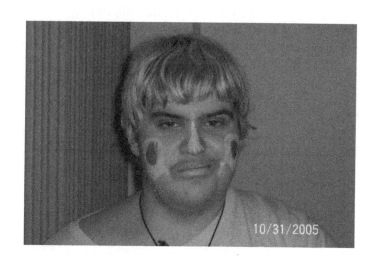

Chapter 3 – The Journey

Being 16 years old and 799lbs pretty much felt like a hopeless situation for a teenager. Life was a drag for me. Kids my age were hanging out with their friends, chasing girls, getting into trouble and enjoying life. For me, however, it was a different story. I was always inside looking at the fun that everyone else was having outside. I remember my friends going for a hike or going outside to play football, and I couldn't because I was too big. It was certainly a life that felt unfulfilled.

Truthfully, I wasn't always morbidly obese, although I was the kid who was always bigger than most of his classmates. I remember in kindergarten I was roughly double the size of most other kids in my class. My peers loved me because I was the bigger kid. By 2nd grade, I was weighed in at the nurse's office at 210 pounds. I remember the nurse looking at me and telling me that was a huge amount of weight for such a young person. They sent home an obesity paper for my parents to read.

Gym class wasn't much fun for a fellow my size. I was slower than everyone else. I didn't have the skill, the speed, nor the desire to even be in gym class. My favorite activity in gym class was dodge ball. I'd stand against the wall in the back to purposely get out because I didn't want to play anyway. I hated going into the locker rooms and being self-conscious about my extra weight. I'd change in the bathroom and wouldn't even want to be around anyone with my shirt off. There were many awkward moments being so large.

Middle school was like a whole new ugly world. All those hormones started kicking in. Everyone seemed taller and bigger. Voices became deeper. Classmates who used to look like ants compared to me shot up to about my height. No longer was I the tallest kid in my grade. I was now the kid who was wider than anyone else in my grade. Upperclassman laughed at me and mocked me as I walked in the hallway. Girls would point at me and laugh. They would dare each other to ask me out. It wasn't the highlight of my life, I can tell you that much. Upperclassman would flash pornographic images at me in the hallways, teasing me and saying I would never be with a female. It all felt like a bad dream. When would I wake up? I couldn't escape it. I had to go to school. I remember faking that I didn't feel good, just to stay home so I wouldn't have to deal with the stresses of school. For that day, I wouldn't have to deal with the daily ridicule as I climbed the stairs, not have to hear nasty comments about the size of my back side.

It was all such a struggle. I'm not here to say I wanted to play the part of a victim. I'm not telling this so you say, "poor Justin". I simply want you to understand my history, as it is a part of my story. My morbid obesity really made me feel like a social outcast. I wasn't well liked by most of the kids. Some fellow classmates called me a "scummer". A few befriended me. Still others were just nice from afar. I didn't care so much, until it came time to pick a partner for an activity, which only worked out when the teachers picked partners for me. It spared me from the embarrassment of not being chosen by anyone.

Sitting at the school desks was always embarrassing. I was too large to sit in the normal student desks. I would have to either pull a chair up to sit at the desks, or the teachers would put me at the computer desks. I felt singled out since that happened in almost every class. Fellow students regarded me as odd and a little off. I didn't want to be looked at as such, but I was.

One incident at school stands out in my mind. I was sitting in class and we were talking about healthy eating. The teacher was going over the lesson, then another teacher from across the hall came in and interrupted the class. He began speaking to the teacher who was teaching the class, asking, "What's going on in here? What are you teaching on?" She replied, "We are talking about healthy eating." The visiting teacher pointed to me and joked, "By the looks of that you aren't!" Both teachers smiled and laughed quietly. My face got red and I was really embarrassed. I couldn't wait until the class was over. Truthfully, there was nothing funny about it.

I've developed true empathy for people who appear to be misfits of our society. It breaks my heart to hear about the bullying that goes on in public schools with students. It bothers me to hear about adults treating other adults as scum under their shoes, because they appear different than others, or because they don't have nice things or fancy clothes. The discrimination has to stop. It never solves anything, and it just makes people feel bad about themselves.

One of the ONE STEP NATION projects that's in the making is an anti-bullying campaign. I make presentations to schools, sharing my story and how I was treated in school. I tell how kids called me names like, "lardo, fatty, waddles, freak, loser, scummer," and how I wore those labels for the longest time. The truth is though, we can be set free from our labels. I encourage the children who are labeled. I tell them the truth, that those labels do not define them. We also speak to the bullies and inform them of the damage that they do to others' self-esteem and lives by threatening someone or treating them badly. I teach the principle of treating others the way you want to be treated. I personally believe that kids need called out and challenged to rise to new heights. Without being challenged, they won't see a need to change or even desire to experience change. I believe The ONE STEP anti-bullying campaign speaks volumes to this generation. It's our desire to see less bullying, more acceptance and kinder kids. I believe this is possible by calling kids to something bigger. Live to love. Live to help. Live to put others before yourself. That's how good things happen.

I could write all day about the challenges of school, about the things students said to me and how they treated me. But I believe you get the idea that it wasn't easy, and it impacted me in negative ways. I eventually asked to be home-schooled due to the stress and my desire to avoid being around people. If I could have observed myself from afar, I certainly wouldn't envy my life.

After the years of misfortune in middle school, and before I was homeschooled, I headed off to high school. This was a big step for me. I remembered the transition from elementary school to middle school. What would high school bring? I would soon find out. On my first day of 9th grade I was absolutely terrified. I rode the bus to school and got off in a whole new universe. Taller kids. Masculine kids. Was I at college? Everyone seemed so different. Now I was the short kid that was extra wide! I entered the double doors and walked into the world of the unknown. Kids were blind to me. Nobody even appeared to look at me. I got to my class and I felt completely invisible. I started to like it. I made some friends, and the judgmental attitudes appeared to come to a sudden halt. I started to like high school. I still sat at desks in a different way than my fellow classmates, but I did seem to be more accepted. However, I still felt very self-consciousness. I was still struggling. Would I get a girlfriend? Would I be part of a group and feel accepted? Insecurities plagued my mind.

On top of this, I was always a peace maker. At home, Mom and Dad would have frequent arguments, and I would always intervene to help them make up and apologize to each other. Trying to be the family peacemaker was a lot of stress for a fourteen-year-old. With tension at home and at school it's not surprising that I developed anxiety and panic attack disorders that changed my life forever, and led me to balloon to an unbelievable amount of weight.

Even before middle school, I developed a food addiction. Food became my friend. I remember being upset when Mom and Dad didn't have the dinner table full of food at 5:00p.m. When Mom came home from work, Dad was supposed to have food on the table. I threw fits if the food wasn't ready on time. I had a problem. It was an addiction. I enjoyed the flavor of food so much. When my parents weren't in the house, I snuck some meal replacement bars and ate a few of them as snacks. I made 3-4 sandwiches at a time, just to hold me over until the next meal. I downed a pound of hot dogs and buns all by myself, just because I was bored. I sent my brother to walk down to the local convenient store and buy me several king size candy bars so I could make it until dinner, which was only an hour away. I was a monster, ready to eat anything. I would drink soda after soda, just to enjoy the flavor. I wasn't thirsty, I was just addicted to the flavor. Mom and Dad bought sub sandwiches almost every Friday, and I often ate a two-foot sub sandwich, all on my own, plus four to five handfuls of chips on the side, along with a few bites of the sandwich that my brother didn't finish. I enjoyed the taste of food. I got lost in it. Every time I took a bite, it made me feel lost in the moment, with no thoughts about my problems.

    I could eat a box of cereal in one sitting, along with a few glasses of orange juice. I shoveled down a huge cake, all by myself. I ate a double cheeseburger, with a normal cheeseburger on the side, followed by a large milkshake and extra-large fries. I was the guy who sneaked snack cakes under my pillow at night, and while everyone was sleeping, I'd get them out and eat a few packs of them. I was like a ravenous bear that was preparing for hibernation. Anything and everything looked too good to pass up, except for lima beans. Somehow, they didn't appeal to me.

    I didn't recognize that I had a food addiction until it was nearly too late. It's amazing how you don't recognize a storm rising until it is upon you. It was as if I was blind to myself and to my food addictions. To me, felt as if my life was normal and that there was no problem. Sure, I was overweight, but I didn't know it was because of food addiction. I was like anyone else. I enjoyed food. So what if I kept eating just to enjoy the flavor of food, no matter how full I felt? It didn't register until I was in the hospital bed in Pittsburgh. It wasn't until doctors told me that I weighed 799lbs. That was a jaw dropper. That was my wakeup call. Obviously, I had a problem. I needed help because I couldn't fix it alone.

    My parents did try to help me shed unwanted weight. My Mom was always a bigger lady herself. She was always trying to lose weight. She tried diets and new ways of eating to help her lose weight. She introduced me to a few different diets that she thought would surely help me lose excess weight. I remember the low carb diet. I did end up losing weight on that one, but I gained it all back, because I got tired of not eating bread and other tasty foods. I tried a yogurt diet, where I ate yogurt for breakfast and snacks, and a normal lunch and dinner. That lost its luster after the third day. I ate too many for it to be effective. I even tried an apple cider vinegar strategy. The vinegar was in pill form, supposedly to help me burn fat, but it never worked. Mom and Dad tried meal replacement bars, and I enjoyed the flavor too much to just stop at one bar.

My parents even tried taking me to a dietician for advice. The dietician gave me some dietary advice that could have really helped me change my way of eating. At first, I followed the guidelines, but then lost interest. It didn't appear that anything was working for me. To be honest, I just didn't give anything a chance to work. I developed boredom from eating the way others prescribed me to eat. I even tried taking metabolism enhancers to help me with energy and fat loss. I tried those for a few months, and they did not help. All they did was keep me up later at night and give me a buzz of energy. Nothing that I tried worked. I didn't know balance. I had a hard time eating in moderation. I had a hard time putting food down after feeling satisfied. I was hooked on food.

With all these issues, you can see how my journey was one of frustrations and hopelessness. I believe a lot of people are in the shoes I was in. You may be reading this book and thinking that you can relate. You may be reading my story and it's reminding you of a spitting image of yourself. I have to say, I've talked to a lot of people with the similar struggles. The good news is that you are not alone. Countless times I've discussed the issues of weight loss with people, and they all have some pretty common experiences. Food addiction is an issue for most overweight people. Not knowing where to start is another issue. Some have no drive to change. Others are just overwhelmed and wish they could just find a method of eating that works best for them. They don't want to try a new diet or a new exercise program. They just want to see change by finding something practical.

    I've been in the shoes of those who can relate. The addiction thing is not easy to break. Food has been consuming us instead of us consuming it. It's time to stop that and it's time to put food into its rightful place. We don't have to be enslaved to a substance any longer. It's time to be set free and it's time to take action. Losing weight is never easy and it can take many attempts to see success. Just know that it is possible, and you don't have to remain stuck in a rut. I look back at my life, and I see the times when I have allowed food to consume me. I was seduced by the comfort, pleasure and flavor sensations. But know that this addiction can and will destroy you, friends, unless you take action. If you examine your life at this moment, do you see food as something that you are enslaved to? What are you going to do about it if the answer is yes? Will you continue down the same road with the same broken results? Or will you take action and recognize the reality that is in front of you? Overcoming addiction starts with recognizing the problem. Are you a person who just doesn't know where to start? When will you finally reach out and get the help needed to see success and transformation? Don't be like me, and wait until it was nearly too late to do something about your weight and your health. We have people in our lives that care about us. You may have children, family, friends and even co-workers who care about you. Why not take action to stick around for them?

    I am not asking you to do something impossible. I am simply calling you to action. Let change begin now. Put down the donut. Get the thought of junk food out of your head. It's time to learn how to be healthier. It's time to apply healthy choices to your life. It's time to take the ONE STEP needed to see change and improve your quality of life. I am thankful that I decided to seek my transformation. God truly opened my eyes to the path of destruction I was on. I was rescued from the storm that I found myself in. I was out of control. Today, I have control. Now it's time for you to gain control. At the end of this book, there's an opportunity for you to seek transformation, ONE STEP at a time.

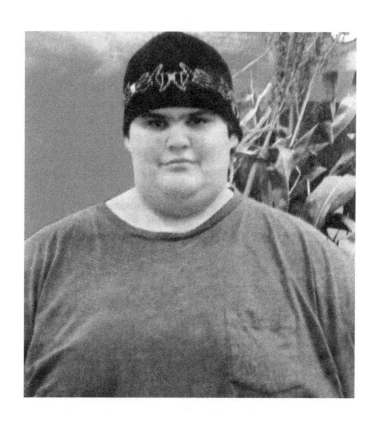

Chapter 4: THE SET BACKS

It wasn't easy to drop 600lbs. As I sit here and ponder the easy days and hard days, there were days when I just simply felt like giving up. It was tiring. It was difficult. It was inconvenient. It wasn't in any way appealing to stick to a lifestyle of losing weight. It required me to stay consistent. It required me to refuse the foods that I'd grown to love so much. It forced me to try new foods that I'd never acquired a taste for. In all honesty, there were days when it was miserable to be attempting any type of weight loss.

It all started in the hospital. I was told I had to move before they would let me go home. By moving, they meant I had to stand up and start walking. That was going to be interesting. I didn't even know if I had the strength to do so. Even maneuvering into a new position on my hospital bed was a challenge that left me winded and forced my heart to beat faster. One day they sent two beautiful nurses in to help me walk. That was embarrassing. I wasn't happy with how I looked, and now there were two pretty nurses who wanted to help me walk. I got out of bed, trying to be macho. I remember the cramping that started in my legs and in my back. I played it off like it was nothing. We walked about 50 steps and I had to sit back down. What a relief it was when I sat down! Though this wasn't so much of a setback, it was still a very hard moment for me. Many people see these moments as impossible. I did have a new faith, and I do believe it gave me a new focus. I don't even know if I'd even attempt a huge obstacle if I didn't have my new mindset. Can an embarrassing moment be setback for some? Possibly. But for me, I wanted to go home. I wanted to see change. I wanted to walk a new path to a new life.

Coming home from Pittsburgh, Pennsylvania was a moment I wish I could forget. They strapped me in for the ride to get home. I remember being about two hours into the ride home, and I had to go to the bathroom. I was too embarrassed to say anything, being so self-conscious, so I just went. I didn't ask for a urinal. I told the paramedic that I had wet myself, and he understood. It was a very uncomfortable ride home. I share that story to tell you that setbacks are real. Though I felt like I had purpose and meaning, I still felt totally insecure. This was something God would have to work on as I drew closer to Him.

At home, I was helped back inside my room and quickly sat down in relief from all the stresses and mayhem that I had just experienced. It was time for me to receive personal care from home. Visiting nurses and physical and occupational therapists came to help me recover. This was also a new experience for me. I didn't want people interfering with my life. I was a stubborn teenager. At first, I was reluctant. I eventually gave in and allowed them to help me. If I didn't let them help me, I may have never recovered. I had to overcome my stubbornness and my pride. I wasn't allowed to be the stubborn teenager who just wanted to be left alone. I needed to be the person who became humble in order recover. The setbacks in my mind certainly challenged me.

Soon after I came home, I recall sitting there and hearing a knock on the door. A few men dressed in blue came in with a big machine. It looked like a big tank from the back of semi-truck. They brought me oxygen to wear. They also brought a compressor that I would be using for what seemed to be forever. They put me on four liters of oxygen at a time. I hated wearing the hose in my nose. It was uncomfortable over my ears, and it made my nose feel dry and raw. I had to wear it so I could get enough oxygen into my lungs. I always felt like I was attached to a leash when I wore the tube. Without wearing it, my oxygen levels went down to 68%. When it was low it was hard to breathe. I had to get used to it, if I wanted to see myself recover from this mess that I got myself into. I just couldn't wait to stop using it.

    I began my journey of getting active again the next day. Two wonderful ladies were sent my way to help me recover. I now had a physical therapist and an occupational therapist. Both of them were a true blessing, and both of them were Christians. It seemed as if God had sent them my way to encourage me and help me. I began building friendships with them, which certainly helped me with my journey. My first setback happened during one of my first physical therapy appointments. My PT asked me to take 50 steps out to my living room from my bedroom. That seemed like an impossible mission. But I was encouraged and inspired to try, so I stood up, and shuffled through my hallway. My family lived in a house trailer, not the roomiest place to exercise. I began walking awkwardly down the narrow hallway, but I had to slightly turn sideways, or else I would not be able to fit. After taking a few steps, out of nowhere, my foot went through the weak floor. I almost fell, but my parents and therapist held me steady. My dad managed to help me maneuver my foot out of the floor and back onto solid ground. I continued the trek to my living room where I collapsed on the couch, breathless. Though I was hoping for relief, I was wrong. I was hit with intense pain in my right leg. I developed a huge cramp from that short walk. The pain was horrendous and I couldn't move very well to position my leg for relief. I sat there in immense pain for a few minutes, trying to massage the cramp out of my leg. This was exhausting! How on earth was I ever going to get past this? I could hardly walk. Somehow, I found the strength to walk back into my bedroom where I stayed the rest of the day. I was informed that I needed to start moving in order to lose weight and get healthy. How on earth was this going to happen? I could hardly walk 50 feet. My therapist left me with some daily exercises to accomplish in order to see results. Let's just say these were not much fun.

With all the visiting nurses and other health professionals coming into my home, I heard a lot of interesting things. One professional told my parents that people my size usually don't live. "That's just great," I thought, "that's what I really wanted to hear." I needed hope, not hopelessness. Talk about the possibility of death scared the living daylights out of me. Numerous times I had mental setbacks when the fear of death ran through my head like an intruder, awakening those negative thoughts. I had to remember that I needed to do something different, or I would die. I had to remember that if I lived or died, I was going to be with my Heavenly Father. I had to shut out fear. I didn't want it to control me any longer. I couldn't allow mental setbacks to become my reality. I had to refocus. With my new-found faith and a will to succeed, I started taking my life seriously. I wasn't about to go down without a fight.

As I began to lose some weight, I began to feel better about myself. I gained strength in my mind, body and spirit. I was feeling like a new person. However, I did experience a lot of discomfort. I developed "big people" problems. I started chafing and it made walking very uncomfortable. I started getting boils between my legs where my legs were rubbing together. It was such an obstacle. I didn't need extra hindrances in my way. It was already hard enough to get moving. Those little obstacles slowed me down a bit, but I was grateful to have a good team of nurses that helped me out.

    On top of trying to recover physically, anxiety attacks continued to haunt me. The exhausting grip that fear of death had on me kept me on the medicines. Though I had a new faith in Jesus, and though I had peace that I never experienced before knowing Him, I still was struggling. Some Christians would say that makes me weak. I say that makes me human. I am not a supernatural being. I am person who is imperfect and in need of a perfect God. I was learning to trust in Him more than anyone or anything else. I don't judge those who are struggling, I empathize with them. I know it's not fun having anxiety attacks. I know the bondage that fear keeps you in. There were times when I was trying to get my steps in, and I would be plagued with them. I knew what they were, but I was still gripped with fear. I couldn't wait to be set free from them. Not being able to breathe from being so overweight was enough of a struggle all on its own. I didn't want to be struggling with two major problems, but I was. Panic attacks took my breath away. Occasionally, I had a panic attack while I was walking around my home. When those moments happened, I wondered if I was going to pass out or keep going. I thank God that I never passed out. I just kept pushing through.

    As I began to lose weight, it got generally easier to function. However, the size of my legs was a barrier to my progress, making it terribly difficult to move freely. They were big. I had huge hard spots of fat and water on my inner thighs; they felt like basketballs, which made it hard to keep my balance as I walked. My legs seemed to take forever to get smaller and lose the uncomfortable spots. Eventually they did end up shrinking, making it easier to get moving.

As I attempted to gain strength, my confidence grew. I began to stand up and walk on my own. I began to try to accomplish tasks without asking for help from anybody. One setback, though, was my balance. Often when I tried getting up, I fell face down on the ground. I could not get up on my own. I needed help. So, I had my brother pile up mattresses in order to give me leverage to stand up. This happened several times, due to my balance being so bad. Even today, my balance is not the best, but I do what I can to make it work. It does prohibit me from doing everything that I want to do, but it's a lot better than it used to be.

There were other setbacks on my journey. At one point, I decided that I wanted to quit and no longer lose weight. I was too tired and it felt like it was just too much effort to keep going. I wanted to be a normal person. Normal people played video games, hung out with their friends, partied, and enjoyed time on Myspace. Nevertheless, I stuck with it. Another time, after I had lost 350 pounds, I took a season off and gained 50 pounds back. Once I had lost enough weight to venture out in public, there were numerous mishaps when I broke people's beds by sitting on them, their furniture and even restaurant chairs. There were many times I was singled out by requiring special seating, such as at movies, plays or concerts. I was frequently the public oddity when I went to stores and places to eat. I felt like a member of the freak show when I was out trying to walk and just be normal again. Kids and adults would stare, and it was all very uncomfortable. If I had let them, social embarrassments would certainly have set me back and made me want to give up and quit.

Thankfully, it wasn't all discouraging. There were plenty of times when I allowed victory to happen instead of defeat. Again, it all comes down to how we view our situations and circumstances. I knew that in order for me to see any type of success and difference, I had to have a different outlook on life. If I chose to focus only on my issues, I would have developed a quitter's attitude and would have thrown in the towel. The old me would have done that. If one bad thing happened, I wanted to just give up and do the easier thing. But, doing the easier thing would never help me. Staying the same would just keep me locked inside a cage of hopelessness. It's so important not to allow setbacks to, well, set you back. Allow them to motivate you. Learn from them and let them become a testimony about how you stood in the face of adversity. Use your story to inspire others, to bring hope to others in a hopeless situation.

One of my early challenges was facing the lofty goal of walking one mile. It felt like an impossibility. I could have abandoned my goal right away, but I really wanted this victory. Truthfully, it wasn't impossible but it was exceptionally difficult. My PT encouraged me to track my progress by keeping a chart. The distance from my bedroom to the kitchen, back and forth forty times, was equivalent to one whole mile. At first, I didn't know how I could complete that task, especially with the discomfort of weighing nearly eight-hundred pounds. Picture holding something that weighed you down so much, that it was hard to even move. My own body weight was a prison that restricted my mobility. I couldn't get it to do what I really wanted it to do. My physical therapist encouraged me to put a penny in a jar every time I made it to the kitchen. As soon as I got to 40 pennies, I had roughly traveled one whole mile. I set my sights on accomplishing that task. It didn't take me one day. It didn't take me 7 days. It didn't take me 12 days. It took me exactly 33 days to complete my first mile. My physical therapist was impressed, and she praised me for doing a good job. I was so excited that I met my first goal, that I began my next mile right away. The second mile took 23 days to complete. After I completed that mile, I started the next one. The next miles took fifteen days, then eight days, and finally, after three months, I was able to walk one mile in one day. I was well on my way; nobody could stop me now. I finally had momentum! I was very thankful for my physical therapist. She encouraged me by quoting Bible verses that gave me confidence, motivating me to finish what I started.

Eventually, my body adjusted to the routine of daily walking. I was up for a new challenge. I was going to walk 10,000 steps. I was going to do this in one day. I tried to mentally prepare myself for the challenge and set a date for the attempt. When the day arrived, my parents and I loaded into the van and set out for the local Wal-Mart. There is no other Wal-Mart for many miles around, so everybody in the whole region went there regularly, though I had not been there for a very long time. My strategy was to walk laps inside, around the store, counting the first lap in order to calculate how many it would require to reach 10,000. With my oxygen tank in hand, I set out, silently counting, my will determined to accomplish the mission. There was no going back. I began walking at a normal pace. People watched and stared as I walked by. I made it through one lap, which was roughly about 900-1,000 steps, therefore,

I had about 9 more laps to go. I started to feel tired and drained after I completed my 2nd lap. I was sweating like I was running a 5k. It was time for lap three. I continued onward, taking it one step at a time. Part of me didn't know if I could do this or not. Negative thoughts crept into my mind, such as, "What am I doing? Why am I even trying to do this?" I quickly threw the negative thinking out of my head and pushed through. My heart was beating fast, my head dripping with sweat. People were looking at me like I was a freak of nature. What did I have to lose? I was tired of defeat. I wanted to see results. I wanted to fix the mess that I had made of myself. I knew that with God, all things were possible. I kept moving. I didn't allow the obstacles of discomfort and embarrassment to threaten the outcome of my personal challenge. Finally, I made it to my last lap. I was wobbling and very sore, my hips were throbbing and my legs were dripping with sweat. My back felt like it was being ripped out of my body. I silently cheered myself on; "I have to do this, I can't quit now. I'm on the home stretch!" When I was about three hundred steps away I focused my eyes on the end like it was a marathon finish line. At that moment, the setbacks didn't stop me; they actually frustrated me enough to want success more than anything. I wanted to move forward. Quitting would never help me progress. It would have been okay to walk three laps around the store, but instead, I wanted more. For the first time in a long time, my personality was coming back. I felt my former competitive drive rise up and break free from its cage. Slowly, but with renewed determination, I walked the final one hundred steps. I could finally taste success. I approached the final step and took it with pride. Incredible! I felt as pale as a ghost, and as sweaty as a marathon runner, but I did it.

What an accomplishment for a person my size. I bought a candy bar to celebrate. It had been so long since I went through a checkout line. Some may wonder why I chose a candy bar. I was so exhausted and I completed such an intense task, I just wanted a treat. I was at a place where I could eat one and not over indulge myself. I climbed into my parents' van, exhausted. It was insane how tired and fatigued I felt. I couldn't wait to get home to lay down. I couldn't wait to tell my therapists about my accomplishment. When I shared the news the next day, they were thrilled with my success. I was sore and still tired, but it was so worth it.

Receiving support really inspires a person to persevere with good behavior. I had a very good support team helping me through the weight loss process. If you are a person who doesn't have a support group, I recommend you find one. Support groups will give you an extra boost of confidence. We were created to encourage one another. We aren't supposed to live life alone and by ourselves. We are social people. Some of us are introverted and we may not like to be around too many people, but everyone benefits from a friend or two to support your endeavors. Support groups help by offering inspiration and encouragement to move forward. They help in the area of accountability, as well. Also, you can use your experiences to encourage others in similar circumstances. I firmly believe the healing is in the helping. Giving back always makes people feel better; it sure does for me.

My support group was there to pray for me. I called my team when I felt tempted to over- indulge in foods that I knew I wasn't supposed to eat. As I got more mobile, I could walk to convenient stores and purchase junk food if I wanted to. When I felt tempted I called my people and informed them about my urges. They prayed with me and encouraged me not to give in.

    Don't get me wrong. I did have my days with setbacks. Sometimes I allowed the temptation to win. I gave in to eating a whole pizza by myself. I gave in to buying cookies and a large cappuccino. I was not a perfect person, by any means. But when I took my health seriously, and had my eyes focused on Jesus instead of myself, that's when I was a better person. That's when I fell less and was able to resist temptation. God promised that He will not let me be tempted beyond what I can handle. I knew I didn't have to say yes to food. I knew I didn't have to say yes to sitting and being lazy. My challenge to you is this. What setbacks are you allowing to rule your life? Identify them and find a support group to hold you accountable. Be transparent about your life. Tell them your struggles. Tell them what they could be praying for. Tell them what they can encourage you in. Give them your number and tell them to text you to check in on you. If you don't receive a text from them, make sure you text them and tell them all is well, or that you are struggling. You were made for more than just concerning yourself with the community of me, myself, and I. Don't allow setbacks to control you. Take one step to overcome them, like I did.

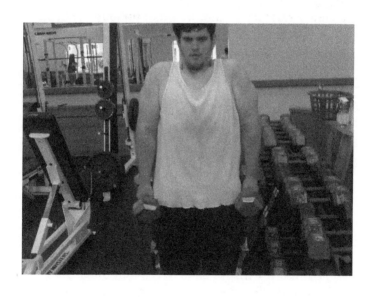

Chapter 5: I'm Alive Again

As I was losing weight, I started to find new ways to challenge myself. I became a member of the local YMCA in Bradford, Pennsylvania. I grew to love that place. I loved walking on the treadmill. I loved lifting weights and seeing my strength increase. I loved going to the sauna to sweat off the excess water weight. I was finally feeling free from what I had become. I felt like a champion that nobody could stop. I was undefeated. With my faith, I found a new sense of purpose. I was experiencing victory over the struggles and addictions. I was excited to be in front of people again. I was finding fulfillment in my life. I was on fire and it felt like I was alive again!

The YMCA was a great place with great support. I went almost every day, religiously. I grew accustomed to the treadmills. Every time I went back, I challenged myself to walk a little further. I started out strolling a few miles, then worked my way up to a brisk three-mile walk. I got to point where I added an incline. Finally, my treadmill workout got boring and stale. I decided to try an elliptical trainer. The first time I tried it I could only stay on the machine for one whole minute. I wasn't used to the motion or the resistance it offered, which was a good thing. My body needed a challenge to see more results. I worked my way up to five minutes, then ten minutes, thirty minutes and finally, one whole hour. One day while exercising, I met a man who used the elliptical like a real athlete. His name was Tom. Tom and I grew in our friendship because we both had goals to lose weight and get healthier. Tom would sometimes go an hour our more on the elliptical machine. One morning I spotted Tom on the machine again and asked him how long he was planning to go. "Two hours today, buddy," he replied. I was taken back, a bit, because two hours of constant exercise was a very long time. I told him I would join him. I was feeling alive and nothing was going to stop me. I latched onto the idea of going two hours on the machine without giving up. Tom and I kept at it for an hour then kept going. The second hour was tiring but I wasn't going to let that stop me. I slowed it down a bit and continued through the next hour. After we finished, Tom and I congratulated each other and shook hands. We were both a sweaty mess.

All the exercise really sparked my metabolism and my weight loss began to pick up. Pound after pound started dropping off right after the two-hour elliptical session. My increased mobility opened up new methods of working out. I was doing an hour of cardiovascular exercise five times per week. Each day I used a different speed, different resistance and different machine. Variety keeps your body from getting use to the same old thing. I don't recommend going all out right away. I recommend making sure you listen to your body, so you know if what you are doing is too much to handle. In most cases, your body can handle more than you think it can. However, if you have a health condition or some type disability, you may want to take it easy and get doctors approval before you start anything to strenuous.

As I began to lose more weight, I began to get noticed by the local YMCA staff. They were very supportive and took the time to talk to me and build a friendship with me. Chuck, the executive branch director of the Bradford Family YMCA at that time, was very intrigued by my weight loss effort, and he decided to call the local newspaper to write an article on me. The Bradford Era featured a front-page story about my successful weight loss of 400 pounds. This opened up a whole new avenue for me to share my story and continue on a successful path.

Suddenly, I was a local celebrity of Bradford, Pennsylvania. This made many people happy about my success and many people became very supportive, contacting me to encourage me. Of course, my small-town fame also made some people jealous, and critical of me and my family. All I can say to those people is this. I've never been an attention seeker. My heart and intent was never to become something spectacular or even a person who was recognized. I simply wanted to lose weight and live longer. But recognition did open up doors to share my story on many platforms. For the record, I am nothing special. I try to take a humble posture at all times. I never consider myself better than anyone else and I pray for success for any person who is looking to make changes to their health. Never in a million years would I want pride to interfere with the platform that God has given me. To those who became jealous and unsupportive, all I can say is, I hope you will come to understand the real me. I am simply a servant of God, a normal person. If I have communicated anything different than that, I apologize.

I was thankful to Chuck and The Bradford Era for writing about my story. I started receiving phone calls from Buffalo, NY television news channels. They came out to interview me and followed my story. This was such an incredible opportunity. I was very excited. Here I was, a kid who used to feel like he had no purpose or direction, suddenly having an opportunity to share hope with others; it gave me a renewed sense of purpose and direction. I felt as if

God was taking the harm I had done to myself and turning it around for the good. I was given a platform to show the world that God saves, and has the power to completely transform a person. My new purpose was to give people hope. The reality is that there are a lot of broken, hurting and lost people. I was one. I am thankful I collided with love and love changed this heart into something special. It's as if I was dead, and now I am alive.

    The *Buffalo News* team traveled two hours to Bradford and did their recording at the Bradford Family YMCA. They aired the piece on their station the following day. I was impressed with their work and I was thankful for the opportunity to share my heart and my story. If it helped just one person, I was satisfied. Little did I know this would enlarge my platform to something even bigger. Soon after the TV story, I started getting phone calls from new reporters across the nation, no longer just the *Buffalo News*. I received a phone call from Diane Herbst of <u>Teen People</u> magazine. She asked me questions about my story. She was really impressed about my successful weight loss, and she wanted to write a story on me. I got extremely excited! I couldn't wait to share my story nationally. She came to Bradford to interview me and see for herself the changes in my life. The story was published quickly thereafter, and it started a flood of responses. People began contacting me via Myspace, telling me that I inspired them. It felt good to be a person who was representing positive change and purpose in life. I didn't want to act like, "poor me - look what I've been through." I wanted to shine light in the dark places. I was a slave no longer. Everything was new, including me. I wanted the world to see that.

At the time the article in <u>Teen People</u> was published, I had lost about 500 pounds. I still had more to go. I decided to step it up a notch as I continued on my weight loss journey. Some great things came about from my connection with <u>People</u>'s Diane Herbst. She had a connection with Dr. Barry DiBernardo, a plastic surgeon in Montclair, NJ. He was impressed with my story and wanted me to schedule an appointment with him. My parents helped me make the appointment, and we went to NJ to visit him. Dr. DiBernardo is a great man. He is very kind and humble. He is very good at what he does. He was interested in helping me get rid of some excess skin so I could move better. When I informed him that I did not have funds for the surgery, and he decided to donate his time and talent to me, because he believed in me. I was very grateful. Dr. DiBernardo scheduled my skin reduction surgery. Meanwhile, the TV show *Inside Edition* wanted to do a piece on me, including Dr. DiBernardo doing the surgery. They came and filmed me before and after the surgery. What a great opportunity to show the world what transformation can look like. I was becoming a new person! I was no longer the self-conscious, intimidated kid that I use to be. I was brand new, and the transformation was happening right before my eyes.

    Dr. DiBernardo offered me several other skin reduction surgeries to help remove excess skin. My family traveled three times to his center, New Jersey Plastic Surgery and Medspa, at 29 Park St. in Montclair, NJ. Each trip was a major undertaking, since it was a six-hour drive. My family was very supportive of the surgeries, even though it was hard for them to come up with the money to make the long trip, stay in a motel, and wait many hours to hear about my condition while I was under the knife for 8-9 hours at a time. It was not easy for me, either. Even with my faith, I had some fear of death, as is always a risk of surgery. Prayer helped see me through my anxiety. Each surgery went really well. He is a great doctor who knows what he is doing. I will be forever grateful to Dr. DiBernardo for his remarkable generosity. I'm so thankful God brought him into my life to restore my physical body.

After the surgeries, I began to feel like a normal person. Over an eight-year period, I lost 600 pounds, through diet, exercise, physical and occupational therapy, skin reduction surgery, and faith in God. I am so thankful for life and for what God has brought my way. One thing I was learning though, was that God is never through with me. If I thought that the journey was over then, I had another thing coming. The hand of God was still at work, even more than I could foresee. I could see His fingerprints on so many things, in the opportunities and people he had brought into my life. Later on, more doors opened up. I was featured in The National Enquirer for my weight loss story. That opened up doors to other media outlets.

My friend Sally Newton, whom I've known for quite a while now, decided to write an article about me and share it with Guideposts magazine. They liked the article and put it in one of their magazines. I was very thankful that Sally took the time to write that. I got to share a lot about my faith in that article, something the other magazines and media outlets didn't include in their pieces. It bothered me, to an extent. Just because they didn't agree with it, doesn't mean that it wasn't authentic to me. I know what I experienced. I appreciated Sally helping me get my story out there to its fullest extent.

About a year later, my story started going international. A lady from The United Kingdom came to the small town of Bradford, PA to do a piece on my life. Imogen was amazed at my weight loss and wanted to publish my story in a magazine called <u>SPLASH.</u> She did two pieces on me, about 1 year apart. The second time she came to do a piece on me, was when I got married on January 9th, 2009. As a gift to my beautiful wife and I, she took professional pictures and gave them to us. We were very grateful! The blessings of The Lord were evident. I couldn't dismiss them. I was favored by our Heavenly Father, just like we all are. He loves us all very much. I am nothing special. I don't deserve the love that He gave me and the blessings that He continues to pour out on me. This is just who He is. I believe if we all just took the time, we'd see the hand of God in our lives. We'd see the blessings and the good things that He does for us on a daily basis. Too many of us focus on the negative. When we do that, I believe we miss out on the beauty God wants to make by taking our messes and turn them into an amazing story. A story that speaks to others and shows them how much He loves and cares for people. I was a kid who didn't know what it was like to be loved unconditionally. I was 799lbs. I felt awful. I felt ugly. I felt worthless. All that vanished when I came to know my Father. It was more than a religion to me. It was a relationship. Something I longed for my whole life and didn't know it until I found it in Him. As I grew in my relationship with Him, I was able to recognize the gifts, blessings, moments of correction, and moments of growth that He put in my path. I am forever thankful for what He has done in my life. I give him all the credit. My ambition is to make Him famous while

I work in the background. If someone sees Jesus in Justin, then I have done my job.

More opportunities came along in the years following the SPLASH magazine piece. I was trying to keep excess weight off, which required daily diligence. My next goal to was to run a 5k, which I did with the help of my friend, Marne. We trained at the Y, and when race day came, we were ready. Marne took off and left me behind, but I persevered at a slower pace. Though we didn't finish at the same time, we both completed the race. It felt amazing! I had never imagined I would ever be able to run a 5K.

That accomplishment gave me a heart for fitness. I decided to get certified as a personal trainer through the YMCA. Marne and I took the required classes and we both became certified. I started training people at the Y who were struggling with their weight, something I'd wanted to do ever since I lost weight.

Out of nowhere, someone suggested that I send my story to The Huffington Post website. I sent it in, and they featured my story in 2014. It was chosen as the most inspirational weight loss story of the year. What an honor! I thank God that He opened up that avenue for me to inspire other people. Soon after, I received a phone call from both the *Today Show* and *Good Morning America*. Both of them wanted me on their show at the same time, and I could only pick one. I went with the *Today Show* because it was a live piece, and I could share my faith openly and freely, even if it was just for a small moment. They flew me out to New York City, which I loved. New York City was so much fun! I enjoyed the architecture, the people and the great food they have. It was a real contrast from my small hometown.

The show had me on a live segment with a reporter named Susan. She asked me about my story. I was able to tell her about my history and about the hope I have in my life now. I got to share Jesus with over 1 million people who would potentially be watching live, and also the ones who would be viewing it on the Internet. This. Was. Awesome! I was so stoked to be able to share my story and my faith. After the interview, my Facebook started blowing up. I started getting messages from people who wanted to experience change in their lives, as well. I couldn't answer everyone at once, but I did pray for them and I did inspire everyone I could. My new Facebook page, ONE STEP NATION was growing rapidly, just from being on a TV show. I began posting videos, inspiration, pictures and anything else I could post to inspire the people who would be following my page. The doors were opening, and with God's help, I was walking through them.

    As time went on, the media attention began to die down. I actually started getting busier with my life. My new goal was to get my education and become a pastor, another thing I had never envisioned myself doing. However, when I was 14 years old, a friend of my Mom's, Marge, had a dream from God one night. She said one day, I would be a Pastor of a church. I didn't know if that was accurate or not. In fact, I pretty much shrugged it off. But, as time went on, God confirmed through my own desires, the counsel of numerous people and in other ways. To make a long story short, I became an assistant pastor of Open Arms Community Church, in my hometown of Bradford. That did take a lot of my time, and I began to slack a little on exercise and also on the strictness of the food that I ate. Many church events are accompanied by food. Well-meaning people would give me treats. I began grabbing food that was quick and easy for convenience.

    I was backsliding with my diet. Too many times I let compromise after compromise creep back into my life. I made the excuse of, "Just one more time, I'll go back on a diet tomorrow." Tomorrow turned into the next day, and so on. My bad habits were sneaking back in and I realized I needed to get back on track with healthy habits. I set a start date, with the goal to fast from junk food for a full year. No sweets, cakes, pastries, candies and anything else that had sugar, except for fruit. I started off well with the fast. I made it nearly a full year. But after watching others eat it in front of me and craving it periodically, I quit after Halloween. Don't get me wrong. I am not going to blame other people for my choice. It certainly didn't help the situation, though. I am really a weak person by nature when it comes to the temptation of food. I needed that support, but this time I didn't make it a point to communicate that. I just assumed people would understand and know what it took to support me. I was wrong. There's an old quote about the word "assume." It fit very well in this situation.

    Even after fasting that whole time from junk foods, I gained 80 pounds that year. Are you kidding me? What happened? I wasn't even eating junk food. However, what I was doing was eating other foods that turned into sugar. In fact, I was eating too much of them. I still ate pastas and white breads. I still gobbled down hoagies on white bread with a generous layer of extra mayo. The weight returned easily. The problem was, I allowed it to. I became too comfortable. I became too caught up in daily life and neglected my health. Part of me thought that the media attention was over, so I didn't have the additional pressure to maintain my diligent habits anymore. That was the wrong attitude to have. To be honest, I began taking my eyes off the reason I had the platform that I did, and that was Jesus. I had begun to rely on the media opportunities to bring me fulfillment. Did I mention I am human and I have my struggles?

The good news? I worked to get my focus back on the true reasons why I needed to lose and maintain a healthy weight. It wasn't for my glory. It was to show the world what God can do through an average person. So, I began to lose the weight slowly. I dropped about 15 pounds, and then suddenly I received a phone call from *The Doctors* TV Show in California, asking if they could have me on the show. That definitely motivated me to take my weight loss seriously again. I lost another 5 – 10 pounds before they had me come out. My wife and I flew out to L.A., and I had to tell them that I weighed 250 pounds. I'll be honest, not being able to claim a 600-pound weight loss did get to me, because at that point it was down to 550 pounds lost. Not that it truly mattered, because that is still a significant amount. But to me, it was proof that I took my eyes off of what truly mattered. I took my eyes and focus off of God's love, and put my eyes back on the love of food. Isn't it amazing how busy and crazy life gets? It's so easy to get distracted. It was for me. If you are a believer, you need to make sure to take the appropriate amount of time to spend with The Lord. It helps us keep on track, and it helps us keep our focus on the things that truly matter, especially in a world that screams so many distractions.

The Doctors TV Show was a great success, though it wasn't live. I still had a good time with it. I am thankful for the people who made sure I had an opportunity to be on the show. The people who called me were very nice. The hosts of the show were very welcoming and caring. I also appreciate my friends Scott and Sally Newton, for helping pay for a plane ticket so my wife could go, too. They donated a good amount of money for our trip to California. What a blessing. Again, I see the hand of God all over my story. I see the many opportunities that He gave me to represent Him. I pray that I did a good job.

Today, at age 30, I still feel happy to be alive. I believe I have my weight under control. I've been writing e-books and continuing my ONE STEP NATION movement, in order to spread hope and faith to everyone who will hear it. The ONE STEP mentality is very simple and very doable. I believe everyone can relate to it. It only takes one step to overcome anything. My significant weight loss began with one step at a time, in my trailer. ONE STEP NATION is a movement that I hope will get America moving again. In my final chapter, I'll be discussing more about ONE STEP NATION. Technically, it's not really the final chapter. My life is still going. I am super excited to see where ONE STEP goes. I'm full of hope, ready and eager to see what the future holds.

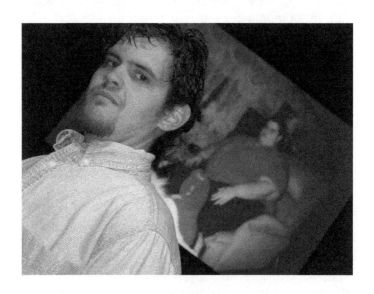

Chapter 6 – The Steps Towards Weight Loss

I understand that as you read this book, you may have some questions about how you can lose weight. I offer a 12- Week program, using proven methods to melt fat and tone the body. The 12- Week program is available at www.onestepnation.com or at www.facebook.com/onestepnation

As I've shared my experiences of catastrophic weight gain and then significant weight loss, you may have some specific questions about how I did it. I would like to give you some details about how I approached weight loss. You have to understand though, that it's not a one -size- fits- all. Really, everyone is different. But I will share with you my step -by- step method of weight loss, Justin style.

Step 1: Mental Preparation

We have to prepare ourselves mentally. I've put together a ONE STEP Small Group Curriculum that deals with mental preparation in more detail. It all starts with the mind, what we believe about ourselves. What we believe about God. All of these matters when it comes down to being mentally prepared to lose weight. Here are seven tips to mentally prep yourself to shed unwanted weight.

1.Determine You Want to Change – Without determining that you want to change, you'll never experience change. You have to make up your mind. This is it. It's either game time or it's not. You have to decide.

2. Write Down and Tell Someone You Want to Change – Do this because it gives you accountability. One of my clients who is a ONE STEPPER, lost 40 pounds by posting on his Facebook page that his goal was to lose 40 pounds. He put himself out there. He even joined my <u>ONE STEP 12 - Week Program</u> and received the extra accountability from me. This individual has seen real success. I am positive that if you write down that you want to change, and make your goal always visible, it affirms your commitment. Tell someone to make it happen.

3. Throw Out All The Negative Thoughts and Beliefs About Yourself – We believe so many lies about ourselves. I know I did. I believed I was unlovable. I didn't believe that I mattered. I didn't believe I had a purpose. But I was wrong. My life has significance. My life has purpose. I am loved no matter what I look like. Since I matter, I need to live my life like I believe that I do. So should you. Destroy all the junk that you've taken in throughout your life. Replace it with truth. That will help you develop your mind into thinking you are worth the time and effort to lose weight. It will help you destroy the lie that you'll be a lost cause forever.

4. Believe Positively and Speak Positively About Yourself – When was the last time you spoke something positive about yourself? When I was 799 lbs, I believed bad things about myself. I remember telling myself that I sucked, and I was fat. When I was okay with thinking those thoughts, I allowed myself to fall prey to mental abuse. Yes, you can mentally abuse yourself. I had to change my thinking. I could no longer allow self-criticism to be part of my vocabulary. If you are a person that does this to yourself, please stop. There's no victory in this. Believe that you matter. Speak out loud that you matter. Speak words of life, instead of death, over your life. Speak the promises of God. Speak the good things you believe about yourself. It will do a world of wonders for your mental preparation.

5. Cast A Vision for Your Life – Without any type of mental vision, you'll have no destination to get to. You'll wander aimlessly, trying to find fulfillment and success. Where do you see yourself in a month? Where do you see yourself in three months? Where do you see yourself in six months, or a year? Get a clear vision and write it down. Go after that vision and try to fulfill it. When you aim for something, you'll eventually hit it.

6. Support Group/Constructive Accountability - I spoke about the importance of this in the previous chapter. If you don't have a support group, you won't see success as easily. All I know is, I've received a lot of help from people in my support network in the form of prayer, encouragement, inspiration, and accountability. All are very important for weight loss success. Developing supportive relationships gives you an open avenue for constructive accountability. Accountability is good for us. We tend to not always want people up in our business, but let me inform you, it will help you become a better person. It's simple. If someone is criticizing you, let them know that they haven't been building you up, but actually tearing you down. You need encouragement and realistic challenges to move in a positive direction; that's what accountability is. If they just don't get it, I suggest finding other supporters.

7. Help Others – The healing really does come from the helping. When your efforts become focused on the good of others, it will also help you stay in the frame of mind for transformation. Giving to others helps you focus and stay on track. People who you help will be counting on you to stay faithful to your progress. It's like this for me. Obviously, if I gained all my weight back, I'd let down the ones whom I've helped. Helping other people has truly given me focus on why I do what I do. I continue to stick to my healthy eating journey, because it not only blesses me, but it blesses others.

Step 2: Learn Food

Food, in general, is a gift. We often look at food like it is an evil substance that makes us fat. That's just not the case. It's beneficial. Food has the ability to help our bodies receive fuel to function normally throughout our day. Natural foods are filled with great vitamins and minerals, proteins, carbohydrates and fats. All are vital for us to consume and for our bodies to function at optimal health.

I had to learn how to eat again. My diet was filled with all sorts of junk. I ate processed foods, white breads, sugary drinks, candy, sugar laden cereals and so much more. I was intoxicated with the taste of food to the point where it consumed me. I became addicted to the flavor. The rich taste of food kept me hooked. I had to learn how to overcome that addiction. I wrote a book called, Food Consumed Me: How I Overcame Food Addiction. It's available at www.onestepnation.com or www.justinwilloughby.com. Reading that book gives you the secrets I used to get past that addiction.

We have to learn that food should never control us. We have to learn that food, eaten in the right amounts and at the right times, it's actually beneficial for us and will help us burn fat. Protein is a major nutrient that we need in order to tone up and even build muscle. Proper protein consumption can actually increase our metabolism, especially if it's partnered with working out. Protein will help you feel satisfied longer.

Fats have the ability to satisfy us. We should include fat in our diet. Trans fats are the fats that we all should avoid. Professionals recommend limiting your intake of trans fats. These fats are not good for your body. Try eating mono- unsaturated fats. Try eating saturated fat in moderation, as well. Fat is not the enemy it was once made out to be. I believe sugar is the greater enemy. When I say sugar, I say sugar from processed junk foods. Donuts, pastries, cereals, candy, etc. These should be eaten in moderation and should not be part of your normal diet. I go in detail about food in the 12- Week Program through the ONE STEP NATION. The 12-Week Program has set people free from their food addictions, and has given them the skills to burn fat by eating properly. Once you learn about food, it will help you understand that it's not the enemy, but can actually be your friend.

Step 3: Learn Activity

When I mention activity, people tend to turn their heads the other way. Activity is usually not fun for people who are trying to lose weight. Some people are afraid to get all sweaty. Others are just afraid of activity all together. We make up excuse after excuse for why we can't exercise or even get active. Isn't it interesting that we will spend hours on our hobbies or watching TV, but we will avoid exercise like it's a plague? Inactivity sabotages your health. Your body was created to move. You weren't created to sit still.

A lot of Americans have a sedentary lifestyle. The rise of obesity and heart disease in our country proves that this is a major problem for so many people. This isn't a slam, it's just being factual. We have to understand what we are up against so we can know how to combat the issue.

When I was growing up, I was never an active kid. I did enjoy playing the occasional football game with my friends, and maybe dodgeball, but when it came to running, jumping and hiking, I wasn't a fan. Lack of exercise led to becoming overweight. Gym class was my least favorite class because it involved activities that I usually didn't like. I didn't want people to see my fat jiggle when I was moving. I didn't want them to make fun of what I looked like in mid run. It was a serious thing for me.

It wasn't until reality sunk in, knowing that I weighed 799lbs, that I knew I needed to do something with my health, and it would take me getting active to do so. My first activity was just standing up and sitting back down, as many times as I could, just to burn calories and get my heart rate up. Sometimes that meant standing up five times in a row and sitting back down. Other early activities that helped me succeed were walking a few steps, and then resting, sit ups while sitting on my bed or using a pedal to pedal my arms. These were activities that I did to help me build strength and get healthier.

Small steps eventually led me to develop a love for activity. I started walking more and graduated to using a treadmill with an incline, constantly tracking my distance. As the treadmill became easier, I increased the speed, the incline and even my time on the machine. As I got used to that, I started using other machines like the elliptical, arc trainer and stair climber. Using weights helped me to build muscle.

Strength-training is actually very beneficial for weight loss. Increasing muscle mass allows your body to burn more calories, even while you are at rest. You're better off exercising using something called high intensity interval training (HIIT), as opposed to a solid hour of cardiovascular activity. HIIT actually gives you the benefits of cardiovascular activity and strength training in one session, saving time and giving you a better workout. Don't get me wrong. I don't dismiss the value of using the ellipticals or stairclimbers, just know that you get better results when you add strength training to your routine. If all you can do right now is walk, that is much better than nothing. By being active in general, you are doing more than half of Americans. You are also doing your health a favor by firing up your metabolism, burning excess calories, building your heart strength, helping to combat cholesterol and triglycerides, and helping to prevent cancer.

Do yourself a favor. Treat your body with respect. Don't abuse it by being lazy and by overeating food constantly. You were created to move. You were created to eat, not to have food eat you. Do what your Creator designed you to do. Do something positive for your health. Understand as you take action to get moving, you are benefiting your body.

I've talked to people who are disabled and cannot run, or even walk. My encouragement to them is to look at life as a blessing. It's a blessing to be alive and your body is still a gift. We can't always escape the results of a world that is broken. Some people are born with physical deformities, or maybe they are injured because of an accident, and suddenly, they may get discouraged, due to not being able to do what everyone else is doing, or not being able to do what they want to do. I say to never let your disabilities control you. You have to control them. Do what you can to get your heart rate pumping. Do what you can to challenge yourself. Do what you can to take ONE STEP to get active. Your ambition will be contagious to those who may be struggling with the same issues you struggle with. Let's be part of the cure. Let's spread hope and encouragement. We aren't victims. We are victors!

Step 4: Life Long Journey

Many people are looking for a quick fix. They look at fad diets and say, "I want to lose weight really quickly so I can look good!" These types of attempts have no substance and often involve unhealthy methods that abuse our bodies and deny them healthy foods, all in the name of attempting to look good. If your reasoning to lose weight is to look good for the ladies, or to have that guy check you out and notice you more, then your reason for weight loss is not valid enough for complete transformational change. If we are led by shallow motivation and fleeting feelings, we won't have a solid foundation for losing unwanted weight. I don't know if you recognize this or not, but our feelings tend to change day by day. One moment we "feel" as if our head is in the game, and suddenly, the next day, we "feel" like we deserve a break. Our reasons to fix our health cannot be superficial, nor can they be because your feelings tell you so. The only way we can possibly lose weight and get healthy for the long term, is to follow through with your deeply held convictions. What do you believe about yourself? What do you believe about your body? What is it that drives you? The birth of victory to overcome unhealthy habits can only come from divine conviction. What do you believe about God and what He says about your body? Changes that are birthed out of conviction are lasting. Just for the record, I am not against wanting to look good. However, we shouldn't find our value, worth or our purpose in our looks. It will drive you insane, and you won't stick with it long-term. If you find yourself in a continual rut of starting out well, but then letting go and quitting within a few days, tired of the same old cycle, you need to come to the understanding that your body is a gift from God Himself, and it deserves to be treated as such. That mindset sets you free. It will guide you into becoming a healthier person. Once a person is comfortable in their own skin, that person will actually take better care of themselves and their body.

    Once you realize that you want to lose weight because of your convictions about your body, you'll want to stick with it. It will become easier to get moving. It will become easier to watch your food intake. You'll understand that becoming healthier is a lifestyle, not a one- time event. Just because you reach a goal, does not mean you give up. Now you have to maintain it. Maintaining is a battle, and it will take lifestyle changes to continue the maintenance phase for your healthier life. It's not a get- rich -quick scheme. It's not a magic pill or formula to make that number get smaller. It's not the traditional American microwave mentality, where everything is quick, painless and easy. It's more of a slow cooker process. It's filled with moments of wins and moments of losses. It's part of growing and making your healthy habits part of your healthy lifestyle. You'll have days when that candy calls your name and you'll reach for it. You'll have days when water just doesn't seem to cut it, so you grab a soda instead. There will be days that you will grab a donut at work, instead of a healthy protein bar. I'm not condoning those behaviors, but I am saying you will fall victim to those setbacks once in a while. When you fall, it's not an excuse to quit and give up. It's an opportunity to recognize your weakness, and try to avoid putting yourself in that situation again. A few mess- ups should never influence your decision to quit. If it's a lifestyle, you won't quit. You'll learn from it and work on ways to overcome it next time.

Step 5: Let your story inspire other people to become a story.

Believe it or not, your story can shine so bright that others will want to live like you. How are you living your life? Do you recognize that people watch you? You may not be able to fathom that, but it's true. People watch us. They watch how we act. They watch and listen to the words that we say. They observe our actions and our interactions with other people. People look for authenticity. What message are you sending to someone who is watching you? Are you leaving a type of legacy for your life that will make others say good things about you when you take your last breath?

I say all this to remind you of your influence. All people have some type of influence on somebody. Kids, family, spouse, parents, co-workers, peers, friends, acquaintances, etc.; your influence matters. It's a shame to be blind to this reality. It robs you and the people around you. Being used as a force for change can really bring a person fulfillment. To be responsible for life change, can really make a person feel good about themselves, and give them a sense of purpose and belonging.

When I examine my life, I see the influence I have on people. I see the spot light that has been shining on me as a blessing. It's one that keeps me in line. It's one that drives me to stay the course. It's one that puts me in a prime spot to be looked at as a genuine influencer or a fake. I preach about a loving God. I preach about weight loss. I preach about health. I am a person who has a voice in different fields. People look at me, as I stand in a leadership position. They will observe me and test me. They will look at me as an example. They will follow me. I speak about eating healthy, but if I always eat junk food, I am just being hypocritical. I preach about Jesus and how He has changed me. If I act like everyone else does, I am being hypocritical. I preach about losing weight. When I don't take my weight seriously, and begin allowing those pounds back, I am being hypocritical.

It's important to understand who you follow, and who is following you. My hope is that people never follow Justin. Justin fails, and he tends to get things wrong. He tends to fall short and be imperfect. Yes, I am allowed to say this, because I don't want to put myself on a pedestal. But when I follow Jesus, it points others to follow Jesus. It's amazing how that works. You become like who you follow. Who are people following when they follow you? How are you influencing others to lose weight? How are you showing people that there is hope and a way to be healthy? Some people are at their wits' end when it comes to their weight problems. They are in a position that I was in, where it is only a matter of time until their obesity kills them. I am thankful I was rescued from that situation. Will you do what you can to rescue others from that end?

Your life becomes a testimony of change once you change. Don't be an example of failure. There's so much at stake. People are suffering from obesity all over the world. It's time for us who have conquered a weight problem to offer hope. I don't hope to get rich by offering a brand-new diet. I'm not seeking to make a million dollars from a new workout. I am genuine and actually care about people. ONE STEP contributes to my livelihood, but it's also the mission of my heart. I really enjoy helping other people. It's not about getting rich. Believe me, if I was in it for that, I would be doing so much more to "make money." My effort is about making ONE STEPPERS. This is about making health important again. This is about YOU realizing and comprehending that you matter. That your story matters. Your experience is one that may benefit others. Stop withholding that from the ears of others and begin speaking it. Be a force of change that this world needs. Taking the step to offer your weight loss or health testimony will benefit you, and benefit others around you.

Now that I have shared my story with you, my hope is that you apply some of these principles to see change for yourself. My latest focus, using my platform ONE STEP NATION, is to provide specific principles that can help others achieve the same success that led to my being able to lose 600 extra pounds. Through my programs, I have numerous tools to guide you towards success. If you need some extra guidance, check out the 7-Day Challenge. Check out my other books. I promise that there are answers for you. You don't need much money to find answers. I'll share my experience so you can experience freedom.

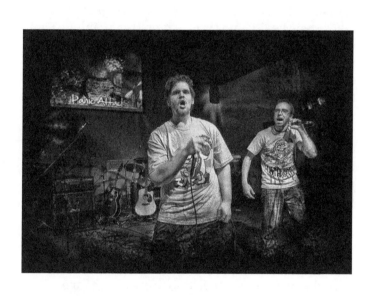

Chapter 7: ONE STEP NATION

Through my story of taking my health back, I am passionate about the same happening for every single person who reads this book, or whoever comes in contact with me. I am not okay with a country that takes their health and throws it out the window. I am not okay with the poor dietary choices that bring on premature disease, poor quality of life and even early death. You were made for so much more than to throw your health out in the trash.

I believe in change. I believe in transformation, starting with the heart. I believe that in order to change in society, we have to begin with changing ourselves. Leaders are often the first to fail. Most people appear to be afraid of failure. Sometimes failing means you did what others wouldn't do, and you learned from it. What if the world's top inventors were to give up after their first attempt at inventing? We wouldn't have the many helpful tools and technologies that we have today. Someone had to pave the way. Someone had to bring the change. Someone had to stay the course and fight in order for their voice to be heard.

ONE STEP NATION is my voice. It's my cry to the unhealthy person who has lost hope in humanity, themselves and God. I deeply care about people, especially the hurting and the broken-hearted. I empathize with others who have had a rough life. I feel for the kids who are bullied, because I was that kid who was made fun of and picked on. I feel for the people who feel hopeless and disgraceful, because they are overweight or obese because I've lived it, and have felt the pain of hopelessness. I long to share with people who are addicted, held in fear, purposeless, because I know that life doesn't have to be lived like that, and there is a way out of it.

ONE STEP NATION is a movement to transform America, one step at a time. It's picked up popularity as media outlets have mentioned it, but it has never been explained properly. In this chapter I'll share what the vision of ONE STEP NATION is all about. Please take your eyes off of me, and onto this movement. I also trust that after you read about it, you'll want to devote yourself to ONE STEPPING.

I picked the ONE STEP motto to make it practical. It's a simple concept to help anyone get better at anything. When you tell someone to take one step at a time, the unrealistic expectations of change happening overnight simply dies. Change is not usually an overnight thing. It's a process. If you have a food problem, it's going to take some time to overcome that problem. I tell my clients to take one step. When you choose a goal, it takes little steps to accomplish it. Once you complete one step, you move onto the next step. It's a simple process and it's one that gives people freedom to fail but still succeed overall. I am not saying that failing is what you aim for. But having the freedom to fail on one small step still keeps one moving forward. Most diets or exercise programs will give very little wiggle room to fail. Once you fail even a little it seems there's no sense of even continuing. That's why with the ONE STEP method, we have you work on one area at a time until you get it right, then you move on. Concentrating on one area will help you master realistic lifestyle changes.

Every good organization has a purpose, vision, mission, value system, but every GREAT organization puts them into practice. Here's ours.

Purpose: We exist to transform the health of individuals in mind, body and spirit, one step at a time.

Vision
The vision of ONE STEP NATION is to seek transformation in mind, body, and spirit of an individual ONE STEP at a time.

Mission: Our mission is to transform lives of as many people as possible by using The ONE STEP Method approach.

Core Values
O – Ownership: We believe that every individual should take OWNERSHIP of their health.

N – No Lost Cause: Every person matters to us. There's no lost cause, only opportunities.

E – Excellence: We treat our bodies with excellence, and we operate in such a manner that exemplifies excellence in our mind, body and spirit.

S – Serving: Healing is in the helping.

T – Team work: There is no "I" in success. Accountability and encouragement is essential for success. We turn successful people into coaches, to multiply our potential.

E – Education: It's important to learn how to treat your body and apply what you learn.

P – Purpose: Purpose is found once you recognize that you exist for something bigger than the temporary. We believe in helping people find their purpose.

Mission of Now

To put the **ONE STEP** core values into practice throughout every aspect of life, including but not limited to, prayer, outreach, decision making, and customer service. In doing so, ONE STEP NATION will teach others how to live life to the full, both physically and spiritually by:
- Teaching/demonstrating approaches for a healthy lifestyle.
- Helping the addicted become set free.
- Helping individuals gain confidence on their journey.
- Informing individuals that they have a purpose and value in this life.
- Offering opportunity for transformation.
- Setting people free from old habits/addictions.

Life to The Full Defined:

To live one's life free from obstacles and burdens that weigh an individual down. To find fulfillment in Jesus and to allow Christianity to mold and shape individuals into living life to the full. (John 10:10)

    Now that you know more about us and what we represent, I have a vision that I'd like to see take place. I believe ONE STEP NATION has potential to go world-wide. It has potential to change the life of any person who struggles with their weight or even addictions. What does ONE STEP NATION offer? Here is a breakdown.

Offers from ONE STEP NATION:
ONE STEP Transformation Program (Justin's Coaching): This is an individually based program specifically designed for you. We give each person a FREE consultation to clarify struggles and goals. We then put each individual through an extensive program full of dietary guidance, a workout/activity plan specifically designed for you to help reach your goals, accountability from other ONE STEPPERS, weekly phone calls with a coach, a once per week Q&A session to help you answer questions that you have with the program or with your personalized plan, and more. This program is designed to give individual results. Our hope is to see transformation in EVERYONE who participates.

9 Week Transformation Course Small Group: A small group curriculum is available for church use and/or home use. The intent of the small group curriculum is to encourage community get-togethers to help with the transformation process. By applying the principles together as a community, you'll be able to experience great success by holding one another accountable. Some of the information given in this 9 - Week Transformation Course is from our 12 -Week Transformation Program. Though it's not individualized, it will help you develop a new mindset. Pairing this with the 12 -Week Program will ultimately give you the best results.

Books: Coach Justin Willoughby has authored several books on health and fitness. Justin also offers books that target individual topics, such as food addiction and successful mindset.

Blogs/Videos: Our blogs and videos are always free. We believe in sharing free information, as it is essential to equip people with the basics of health and wellness. By learning the basics, positive results will be in your future.

Facebook/Website: You can stay updated with One Step Nation with the following.
Website: www.onestepnation.com,
www.justinwilloughby.com
Facebook: www.facebook.com/onestepnation

Public Speaking: Coach Justin Willoughby offers public speaking engagements to schools, churches, health events, community events and more on the following topics: health, spirituality, anti-bullying, self-image and more

Join the movement to see America transformed. I hope that after reading this chapter you will be inspired to join the movement. By joining the movement, you are committing yourself to taking the necessary steps to better yourself. This only happens when we take the ONE STEP that we need to make it happen. Spread the word! Let's get stepping to a better us!

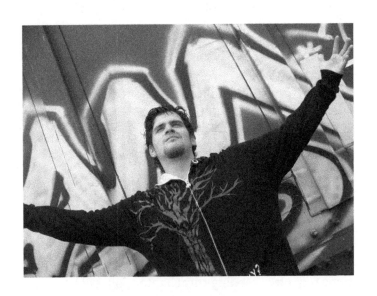

Chapter 8: Your Only Hope

I put this chapter at the end, because I really feel that it brings everything together. This chapter is about faith. Before you close the book, please, hear me out. Some of us may have had a bad taste of spirituality. We may have been wounded in the past by Christians, or at least by people who confess to be. Firstly, I'd like to apologize for the actions of some people who confess the name of Jesus. Jesus told His followers two most important things; love God with all of our heart and then love others. It's pretty simple. Some Christians do not act out of love, and for that, I apologize. If you've experienced this, please don't throw the baby out with the bathwater. Please don't think just because of one bad egg, the whole dozen is bad. I ask you to give just a few moments of your time, as I explain how Jesus became a reality to me. I'd really appreciate that.

I realize that I've saturated this book with all sorts of spiritual words. I've talked about Jesus in every chapter. Why? Because He is the most important part of my life. I believe He gifted me with a new life and a new opportunity to make it right. I don't want to keep quiet about it. Why would I keep quiet about a gift that I've received? Have you ever received an amazing gift, and it was so amazing, that you just had to tell someone about it? That's me. That's how I felt when I wrote this book. I've been given such a gift, and I'd hate to hide it, and I'd hate to not share it with you.

Here is my story. I was never a religious person growing up. My parents never went to church, and we never really talked about God. My Dad would sometimes bring it up, but it was usually in a cuss word or a quick passing conversation. My Mom grew up in church, but she left the scene when she got older. I never understood anything about God. In school, I remember some kids talking about it, but as soon as the teacher heard it, she would end up changing the subject. I remember seeing churches and asking what they were. My Mom would respond, "That's where God lives." I had some type of interest in God, but I never fully understood it. Did He exist? Was there a heaven? Was there a hell? All these questions, but no answers.

One day, someone finally told me about Jesus. Someone told me about the Bible and about church. Someone shared with me how God could help me through my anxiety and panic attack disorder. So, I went to check out a church. I got my family to go, and we started going pretty regularly. I eventually lost interest, mostly because I got too big to feel comfortable to even attend. I stopped going and basically went back to just questioning faith and wondering if any of it was true. Believe me, I've searched. I checked out Islam, Judaism, Spiritualism, and Buddhism. Why would Jesus be any different than these other faiths? What makes Him unique and special?

To be honest, at first I didn't know. I had learned enough to know His story was different. No other God came to earth to die for His people's mistakes. No other God made Himself accessible to us at all times by dwelling in those who called on the name of Jesus. There were a lot of good qualities of Jesus that captured my attention, which no other faith could touch.

It wasn't until I was at my lowest point that I cried my heart out to God, and He answered me. I was willing to put my trust in Jesus and give Him my hurts, addictions, shortcomings, failures, insecurities, fears, depression, weight, and so much more. I didn't know what that would look like. I didn't know how I could do it. I just simply said words from my heart. I apologized for living my life selfishly. I apologized for not caring about Him. I asked Him to forgive me of every wrong I ever committed against Him, and asked Him to be The One in charge of my life. Because, as I observed, being in charge of my own life gave me negative results. It almost killed me.

He did just that. I was willing to take that chance and say yes to God. The moment I said the prayer, is the moment life began to make sense to me. I found my purpose. I found love. I found acceptance. I found answers. I found peace. I found all of that when I made Jesus the priority of my life. I took the trust out of my hands and placed it in His hands. I still struggled with certain things. I struggled with looking at porn. I struggled with fooling around with my girlfriend. I struggled with gossip. I struggled with still having a lot of fear. I wasn't out of the water. I was still in the water, but no longer was the water over my head, drowning me. I was now waste deep, and the water was becoming shallower as time went on.

I began reading the Bible. It was God's words to me. I read it to learn who He is and what He expected of me. I admit, I had some pretty intense questions, because some of the stuff I read, I didn't agree with. Some of the stuff I read, I felt as if God was cruel and mean. Once I pondered and prayed about those things, I began to get answers about why those things that made me uncomfortable were included. It's a long list of answers that I cannot talk about here. I just knew God had reasons. I knew not everything that happened in the Bible was approved by Him, but

He allowed it to happen. I also knew that culture influenced what I read. We read the Bible from an American point of view. His word was written from a Middle Eastern point of view. Certainly, that explains why some things we read strike us as odd. Nevertheless, there is a reason for everything that's in the Bible. When something troubles me, I pray about it, seek answers, and ask wise people, then I receive the answers that I am looking for. Of course, there may not be an answer to every question that we have for God, but that's okay. This is where faith comes in. We know that He is in control and He cares for us as His creation. That's what truly matters.

If it wasn't for Jesus, I wouldn't be here today. If I could somehow change your mind on who He is, I would do everything in my power to make that happen. I do pray for the ones reading this book, that their faith would be fanned into flame or ignited for the first time. Life is too short to allow addictions, cravings and messes to rule us. We weren't created to worship the created things of this world. They are simply gifts for us to use and to enjoy. We weren't made to become enslaved to food, sex, drink, and the like. Substances should never become our god. Addictions might be a flawed attempt to be validated, to cope, or to find comfort. I say Jesus should own that spot. I believe He can set us free from our addictions and our struggles. We tend to think it's impossible, but with God, ALL THINGS ARE POSSIBLE. Why do we limit the Creator of the universe? He is greater than we can ever imagine.

You may be sitting here as a person who struggles with food addiction or some other type of addiction. Today is your day to allow Jesus to take that addiction. You have to allow Him to become your addiction. You may be sitting here enslaved to an extra amount of weight. Today is your day to allow God to help change your mind, to be set free from the damage of obesity. You may be reading this book, and you've been looking for a sign or a moment to find hope and peace. My friend, you've found the moment right now. Don't pass this up. Jesus is alive. Jesus is in love with you. Jesus wants to have a true relationship with you, His child. You are fearfully and wonderfully made. You are loved beyond anything. It doesn't matter what negativity people have said about you in the past. I was called a bunch of names by cruel people. Does that define me? Absolutely not. What defines me is what He says about me. His opinion of me is the ONLY one that matters.

Let today be the day you say, "yes" to Him. Let today be the day Almighty God meets you for the first time, or as a recommitment. God wants to wreck your life. God wants to invade every area and turn you into His masterpiece. If you're ready to give it all over to Him at this moment, I will lead you in this prayer. Remember though, it's not the words that you say that will change anything. It's your words and your heart behind those words. If you mean this with all of your heart, He promises to meet you where you are at. He promises to become your Heavenly Father and your go-to when things aren't going well. He wants open communication with you, His kid. He doesn't want you to think He is mad at you. He doesn't want you think He hates you. He doesn't want you to think you are a lost cause. My friend, you are not! You have purpose. You matter! You were created in His likeness and His image. You were made by God and for God. You are His! He wants you to accept Him as your God. He is jealous for you! He wants your attention. He wants your life. He wants YOU. If you are ready to make that commitment and if you're ready to say yes to Jesus, use this prayer to cry out to God.

Prayer:

Father God, I am sorry for living life my own way and for not caring about you. I've lived as if you didn't exist. I've become addicted to your creation. I have struggles that I need help getting rid of. I am not happy with how I have been living. I need your help. Today I call on Jesus. Today I ask Jesus to be The One in charge of my life. I want to live life your way, and I want to get the results that you have for me. From this moment on, I dedicate myself to you. I accept your example for me. I accept your death on the cross for me and my mistakes. I believe that you rose again from the dead. I believe you are God. Please live in me. Please invade me. Please help me to honor you in everything that I do. From this moment on, you are in charge. In Jesus name, Amen.

Friends, if you said this prayer. I am so very happy that you made that commitment. I appreciate you taking the time to read this book. I appreciate you taking this time to read this chapter. My sincere prayer is that you've experienced hope by reading my story and hearing about My God who has changed my life. I know He can get you through whatever you are facing.

If you made your commitment to follow Jesus today, some steps you should take are.

1. Read God's word. Download *Life Church's* Bible App. It's free and there are many translations you can understand.

2. Find a church home. Hang out with God's people and celebrate what He did for you, and what He is doing for others. You may need to pray and seek out a church. The first one you go to may not be the right fit. That's okay. Don't give up. Keep searching. Find one that preaches God's word. Find one that you can trust. Find one that challenges you to grow closer to Jesus and live on mission for Him.

3. Prayer life. Make sure you talk to Him. To know someone, you have to talk to them. If you got married and never talked to your spouse, would you truly know your spouse? No, they'd be at best, a great acquaintance. Get to know God by talking to Him. You may find prayer awkward at first, but the more you do it, the better you will get.

4. Hang out with Christians. It's important to follow the example set before us. We need to make sure we get with other Christians, so we can get support and accountability. It will help us grow in friendships and our relationship with God.

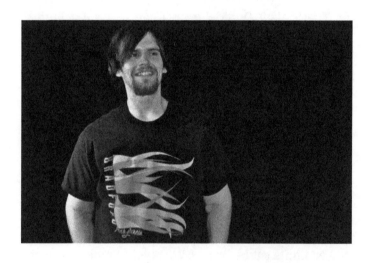

Remember friends, with anything, it only takes one step to get moving and to get started. Be blessed and share this book with others. I'd love to see it reach countless people. Let it inspire America and the world to take their health seriously, and to treat their body as the gift that it is. Your transformation starts with, one step.

- Justin Willoughby
<u>justinwilloughby.com</u>
<u>onestepnation.com</u>

JUSTIN WILLOUGHBY'S
ONE STEP METHOD

A STEP BY STEP PLAN FOR PERMANENT WEIGHT LOSS

JUSTIN WILLOUGHBY

JUSTIN WILLOUGHBY'S ONE STEP METHOD:

A Step by Step Plan for Permanent Weight loss.

Step 1: Make up your mind - 92

Step 2: Mind renewal - 97

Step 3: Erase the myths you've learned about diet/about yourself - 108

Step 4: Food - 116

Step 5: Exercise - 134

Step 6: Accountability/Support Group - 144

Step 7: Spiritual Health – 150

Step 8: Mind/Body/Spirit (Offense and Defense) - 157

Step 9: Celebrate - 163

Step 10: Share your story - 168

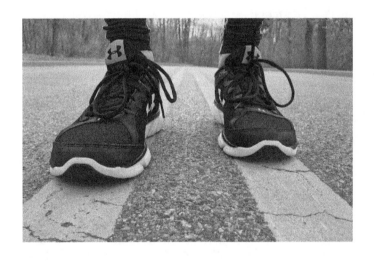

STEP 1: MAKE UP YOUR MIND

We've all had to make a decision that would somehow impact the rest of our lives. Today, I want to share with you a decision that I had to make to impact the rest of my life. Before I begin, I want to share my story with you.

I have always struggled with my weight. In elementary school, I weighed 210 pounds. I gained weight every time I entered a new grade level. The weight gain made me feel insecure. My classmates were all "normal" sized people, and here I was about three times their size. When I hit middle school, the upperclassmen began making fun of me, ridiculing me because of my weight.

One of the primary reasons for my obesity was the fact that I had a food addiction. Food was like a friend to me. I liked to eat when I was happy and when I was sad. When I was made fun of, I would simply eat to numb the pain and embarrassment. It was a vicious cycle that kept me in a constant downward spiral. My addiction continued as I began high school. I was the largest teenager in my high school. I wasn't blind to it; I saw it. I would always wonder what the teachers thought of me. What did the parents of my fellow classmates think of me? My insecurities led me to retreat from the world. After 9th grade, I began to be home schooled. I no longer had to endure the insults, stares, whispers and harsh judgement from others. I no longer had to be concerned about what teachers and parents thought of me. I was on my own.

It was fun to be home schooled, but that didn't stop my ballooning weight gain. I was finally forced to see a doctor, who was alarmed at my condition and arranged to have me sent via ambulance to the children's hospital in Pittsburgh, PA, right away. In Pittsburgh, I got the life altering news that I weighed 799 pounds, and was considered morbidly obese. Doctors did not know if I was going to live or die. It was my ultimate moment of crisis. There I was, a 16-year-old teenager, who may not be taking his next breath. I had so much I wanted to do yet. I wanted to get married. Have children. Find a career. The danger I was in from my extreme weight threatened to snatch away all my hopes and dreams. You can learn more about my story in my book, **ONE STEP: How I Took One Step to Lose 600 lbs.**

Now that you know about my struggle and how I got to a point where I needed to lose weight or die, you'll understand why I have a strong desire to help other people. Ultimately, it's because I almost died. With my ONE STEP method of shedding weight, I'll share how I ended up losing 600 pounds. I can assure you, that if you apply these ten steps to your lifestyle, you too, can lose the weight that you want to lose. Here is step one.

Step one begins with you making up your mind. I am not going to sugar coat anything when it comes to these steps. I am going to jump right in and give you what worked for me. I will share some of the side stories of my life, but if you are interested in more of the personal details of my struggles, I encourage you to read my biography. Making up your mind is ultimately the first step. Nobody can force you to lose weight. Nobody can force you to take a step. You can talk to countless doctors and other professionals, but the reality is this; if you don't want to lose weight, you won't. I had to find the reasons why I wanted to lose weight.

Making up your mind begins the process. First off, I had to recognize why I wanted to lose weight. I was sick of being fat. I also wanted to be around for my family, and to live longer. I challenge people to find some motivating factors to keep them in a mindset for weight loss.

Motivating factors are a huge contributor to success. Often times, it's easy to get your focus off of weight loss. It's easy to just throw in the towel and give up. The question is, what will help you so you don't? What will it take for you actually make up your mind and to stay committed to that decision? I know what it takes. I've been there. Here's some work for you to do right now. Write down up to three motivating factors on the lines provided below. Take a picture of them and make that your cell phone background. Write them on your refrigerator. Put them in your wallet or post them on your bathroom mirror. Place them on your pillow or nightstand. Make it visible so you will not forget why you made up your mind to take your life back.

Motivating factor #1:

_____.

Motivating factor #2:

_____.

Motivating factor #3:

_____.

    Be intentional about keeping your motivators in the forefront of your mind. You may have to repeat these to yourself every day so it reminds you why you are committed to improving your health. Value yourself. You are worth it. Don't take another day to decide. Decide right now. If I would have decided earlier, I would have spared myself the pain of gaining so much weight. If I can help you make up your mind, I will do that. Think of your children. Think of your family. Think of your faith. Now make your decision.

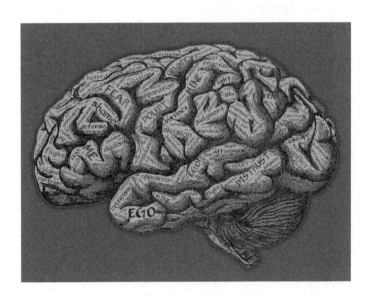

STEP 2: MIND RENEWAL.

We've all developed some bad habits over our years of existence. These bad habits have become comfortable. We've allowed these habits to become a way of life. But truthfully, bad habits should never be normal. First, we need to become aware of the bad habits that are not serving us well.

My bad habits were in the areas of food and activity. I'll share them with you. You may be able to relate to some of them.

Bad habit #1: I became lazy. I allowed laziness to take over my life. I would have my brother get the remote for me because it was too far away. I had my parents make me food when I was hungry instead of getting up to fix it myself. I would ask my parents or my brother to answer the phone so I didn't have to get up to answer it. I even had my friends do things for me. Little did I know that my choices would have a negative impact on my future. Often times the things that appear harmless end up contributing to our long term weight gain.

Bad habit #2: I always wanted to eat until I was full. I did not want to walk away from the dinner table a satisfied person. I wanted to walk away feeling like I just got finished with Thanksgiving dinner. I had a terrible time saying no to seconds. I found myself filling up on foods that weren't good for me. A few extra handfuls of potato chips at dinner. A few extra sandwiches if the main portion at dinner didn't fill me up. I was a machine when it came to eating. I felt like a bottomless pit. I would watch my friends and family barely finish their meal, and I would be on my second or third helping.

Bad habit# 3: Snacks were main course meals. I would eat snacks as if they were meant to make me feel filled up. One candy bar wasn't enough, I needed two. I would buy a king sized and a regular candy bar. It helped me feel fuller and satisfied my desires.

Bad habit # 4: Drinking my calories. I decided that soda and powdered sugary drink mixes tasted amazing. I included sugar laden soft drinks in my standard diet. Little did I know that this would add many extra calories and more ways to gain weight.

Bad habit #5: Not being social was an issue for me. I was the type of kid who did not want to be social. I knew I looked different than other kids due to my weight. I didn't want to end up being laughed at, or made fun of. I would stay in and not go out in public. This lead me to not be held accountable to anyone, and also to remain lazy.

Bad habit# 6: Believing what others said about me. I sat around believing the labels that people put on me. I accepted them like they were a true part of me. I carried them with me as if they were part of my identity. By believing these labels, I fell prey to hopeless thinking. I was stuck in a rut of depending on food to help me get past the negative feelings.

Bad habit #7: Disconnecting from friends. I allowed myself to get disconnected from people who cared about me because I was ashamed of what I ended up looking like. I believed the lie that I could get through this on my own. If I had allowed people to stay close to me, I may have avoided such detrimental weight gain.

Where are you at with bad habits? Part of overcoming those bad habits is recognizing them. Take a moment to admit your bad habits and write them down.

Bad habit #1:

Bad habit #2:

Bad habit #3:

Bad habit #4:

Bad habit #5:

Once you figure them out, you'll need to be intentional about replacing those bad habits with good habits. What are some counter habits that can replace the bad ones? What will help you reach your goal instead of adding to the negative consequences of the bad habits? I have several good habits that I developed over the years to help me lose weight and to keep it off.

Good habit #1: Forcing myself to get active. I make working out a priority. I treat it like it is an appointment that I cannot miss. I try to block off 1 hour per day to exercise. There are days when I have more than an hour, and there are days when I have less than an hour. I am at a place in my life where if I miss a workout, I feel anxious and as if I missed an important part of my day. Exercise could also become a bad habit if not controlled. I understand that life gets busy. I don't beat myself up for missing a workout here and there, but I end up feeling like I missed out on something great if I do miss one.

Good habit #2: Moving every hour has become a must! I no longer can stand sitting for more than an hour straight. I try to get up every hour to walk for 3-5 minutes. This has led me to get up during work to walk around, and even during watching some of my favorite TV shows.

Good habit #3: Prayer has been a huge contributing factor to my weight loss success. I am a firm believer in Jesus and in prayer. I believe my conversations with God can help me stay focused by keeping my cravings under control. A day without prayer with my Savior is a day that I feel lost and neglected. I know that it's not His fault, but mine if I feel disconnected.

Good habit #4: I no longer desire to ask people to do things for me. I force myself to stand up and get the remote. I force myself to walk to the kitchen and get a drink. I even take it upon myself to make dinner for my wife and I. I don't want to fall back into laziness. Laziness nearly destroyed me.

Good habit #5: I have developed a support group. I have people in my life who I can talk to about my temptations, cravings and mess ups. I have a great church family who prays for me, encourages me, and who holds me accountable.

Good habit #6: Memorizing scripture has become a good habit. I choose to believe what God says about me in His word. I memorize His words to me so I can dismiss what the world says about me. My identity is in Him, not what other people say about me. Friends, that mindset is incredibly freeing.

Good habit #7: Tracking the food I eat is a great habit I have developed. Writing down what I consume helps me see what I struggle with, how much I ate, what improvements I am making, or what changes I need to make. Knowing that I will write down whatever I eat or drink keeps me from mindless eating. It's a real secret to success.

    My good habits contribute to my continued success. I set myself up for winning. So, set yourself up for winning by doing what it takes to transform your life. Who you surround yourself with is important. Your choices to prioritize your health will impact you in a positive way. Your food consumption will either hurt you or help you. The secret to success all comes down to you taking the steps needed to overcome the bad habits. Next, I want you to write down five good habits that you can add to replace your bad habits.

Good habit# 1:

Good habit# 2:

Good habit #3:

Good habit #4:

Good habit #5:

Habits matter. Act like they do. Why do we allow bad habits to rule us? Are they worth it? Is the moment of pleasure worth the negative impact on your health? On your soul? On your spirit? Will the choices you make today to feed those bad habits possibly create an addiction? There's a lot at stake. What will you choose?

The next part of mind renewal is to overcome negative thinking about yourself. We've all looked in the mirror at times and been disgusted by what stares back at us. We've all been in a situation when we believed negative things about our looks and our body. We say things like, "If only I could look like that guy or that girl". We may try to find someone who we wish to potentially look like. Maybe it's a celebrity. Maybe it's a friend or a co-worker. We compare ourselves to others like it's our mission to become like them.
Let's take a time out for a second. Stop all the negative noise that is going on in your head, and let's come back to reality. I have a lot of experience when it comes to negative thinking. I had so many negative thoughts about my 799-pound body, that if you heard my thoughts, you'd potentially tear up. It's not okay to think negatively of yourself. You weren't created to hate yourself. You were created to appreciate the gift that you are.

Here are a few spaces to write down the negative thoughts you have about yourself.

Negative #1:

Negative #2:

Negative #3:

     I want you to be aware of what you think about yourself. Really ponder those thoughts that you wrote. Let's think rationally for a second, instead of thinking what we feel about ourselves. Is there truth to the thought? Are you being too hard on yourself? What do others see in you? If you looked deeper, what would you see instead of the "flaws"? Are you aware that your thoughts are making you feel insecure, unattractive, discouraged and unloved? Thoughts have the ability to make or break you. God's word tells us to be transformed by the renewing of our mind.(1) When we stop believing the lies about ourselves and start allowing our minds to be transformed, that's when we see victory.

The next exercise is for you to start your mind transformation. This is essential for you to experience total transformation in your physical appearance. God's word also tells us that what you think, you become.(2) What are you thinking yourself into becoming today? You can use your mind to transform yourself into the person you were created to be. You don't have to think negatively all of the time. You can choose to think positively. In all honesty, what you believe about yourself is a choice. What will you choose? Let's start by choosing to believe good things about ourselves. Write down three positive thoughts that you can use to combat your three negative thoughts.

Positive thought #1:

Positive thought #2:

Positive thought #3:

I encourage you to do what I did. Saturate yourself in what God says about you. Surround yourself with positive people and positive situations. Don't keep yourself trapped in a negative situation. You become what you think. Don't allow yourself to think negatively about yourself. You are a gift. You are a creation of The Most High God. You have value and you have worth. You'll need to truly grasp that, like I did, in order to see total transformation. I promise that if you learn to cherish who God made you to be, you will see evidence of real transformation in no time.

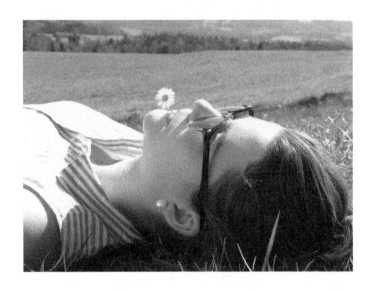

STEP 3: ERASE THE MYTHS YOU'VE LEARNED ABOUT DIET/ABOUT YOURSELF

Myths are everywhere. Myths can be believable if we accept them as truth. Over time, we can allow myths to replace the truth. When it comes to diet and exercise, there are so many opinions out there. Some believe low-carb works better than high-carb diets. Some believe cardio exercise is better than strength training. I am devoting this section of The ONE STEP Method to help you develop the truth for your lifestyle. With so many conflicting diets, what's the best one? Who should I listen to? What's the best way to lose weight? I am here to shed some light on these subjects for you.

Myth #1: One diet works for everyone.

Truth: ONE STEP is not an actual diet. It's a transformation program. It sets you up for success. It's a doable program that anyone in any situation can utilize to help them experience transformation in their health; mind, body and spirit. By applying the steps, you will see ultimate transformation. You will no longer be enslaved to far-fetched diet programs and exercise routines. There is no diet that will work for everyone. Some people have allergies that may prohibit them from following a certain diet. Some people have health issues, and they may not be able to subscribe to a certain diet. Some people have a hard time exercising due to injuries. This will potentially disqualify them from certain workouts. Repeat after me: there is no one- size- fits- all diet and exercise program. This program is about personal lifestyle transformation that will lead to your own success story.

Myth #2: I can't get into shape because....

Truth: A lot of us will look at our situation and believe that we cannot possibly get healthier. We may use the excuse of being too old, injured, confined to a wheelchair, out of shape, etc. I am here to tell you that no matter your starting point, there is always potential to get in shape and to become healthier. The first thing you need to do is find a method of eating that works well for you. Listen to your body. How does your body respond to fats? How does your body respond to carbohydrates? What helps you feel satisfied when you eat? What helps you not get hungry again an hour later? Your body is a blessing. It will let you know what is working and what isn't working when it comes to food and exercise. Are you always tired? There may be a problem with your food selection. Are you always drained? You may need to exercise more. Don't even say that you can't get into shape. If you are able to move and choose your foods, the sky's the limit for you.

Myth #3: It takes a lot of cardio exercise to lose weight.

Truth: This is simply not true. Cardiovascular exercise is important for heart health. I really love doing cardiovascular exercise. But I also know that it's not the only option for weight loss. Walking, running, ellipticals, stair climbers and bicycles are all considered cardio activities. Many people go to the gym and end up working up to doing an hour straight of cardio almost every day of the week. They see some promising results right away, but at some point they experience a stall in their weight loss. They also begin to lose muscle along with fat. Your body is designed to move. There are efficient ways of exercising that burn more fat and increase muscle strength. High Intensity Interval Training is a type of training that you can do to accelerate your weight loss and get the body transformation that you desire. You don't have to camp out on a treadmill every day of the week to see results.

Myth: I can out- exercise a bad diet.

Truth: This is absolutely false. You cannot outrun a bad diet filled with bad foods. You may be able to burn off excessive calories, but you cannot outdo the negative impact some foods have on your body. A diet full of trans-fats and sugary fried foods will ultimately end up causing health problems and obesity. Spare yourself the trouble by cutting down on these foods. Don't rely on exercise to create the transformation you want. Exercise is just one tool to get where you want to be.

Myth: Fat- free is the way to be.

Truth: Absolutely false. America went through a fat-free craze for a period of time. I believe we are finally about to leave that craze behind. A certain amount of healthy fats are necessary for your body. You need fat for a variety of reasons. Fat helps you stay satisfied. Fat is essential for your body to absorb certain vitamins and minerals. When you starve your body of fat, you'll have to replace it with something different. Most of the time we replace fat with sugars. A much better approach is to eat everything in moderation. A healthy amount of fat happens to be essential for everyone's diet. Don't skip the fat. Just mix up your fats: mono-unsaturated, poly-unsaturated and saturated. They all have roles to play in your health.

Myth: Supplements/programs produce miracles.

Truth: Supplements are tools. Some products may help raise your metabolism and erase unnecessary hunger, but there is no miracle supplement. There are so many supplements on the market that promise to deliver the best results. Ultimately though, it comes down to what you do to partner with those supplements. If you use meal replacement shakes you still need you to make healthier decisions the rest of the day. Exercise programs work better by following them correctly while feeding yourself the right diet. It's your choice. There's no magic program/supplement. They are only tools that can potentially be helpful.

Myth: If I don't eat, I'll lose weight.

Truth: This may be true to an extent, but it will eventually catch up with you. Your body needs calories to function. If you starve yourself, your body will begin eating muscle, as well as fat, in order to get the energy needed to survive. There will come a point where your body will slow its rate of calorie burning as it senses potential starvation, making it more difficult to lose weight. You don't do yourself a favor by not eating. You may see some short term results, but it will come with a price. That price is usually your health.

Myth: I don't matter.

Truth: You do matter. Jesus says that you do. Why not believe God? I choose to do that. It gives me a whole new mindset. It helps me understand that I am accepted. I am loved. I matter. To think you don't matter is to think you aren't worth it. You were so worth it, that Jesus went to the cross for you! He said you mattered. Trust that you matter. When you recognize that you matter, you can easily view life through a different lens, a lens that says that you matter. And if you believe that you matter, you will make better decisions based on your value.

Myth: I can't lose weight.

Truth: It may appear to you that you cannot lose weight. You've tried it all. You end up doing well for a few days, maybe even weeks, and then you give in and quit. You feel stuck in a rut. Good news! You can lose weight. You can lose weight by taking the steps to see transformation. Read through the steps and apply them one step at a time. Once you master one, you're ready to move onto the next.

Next, I want you to write down some myths that you believe. Write down the truth below those myths.

Myth:

Truth:

Myth:

Truth:

Myth:

Truth:

Myth:

Truth:

Myths can be replaced with truth. Believing truths over myths will set you free from the prison of lies that you've developed about health and fitness. Let the truth set you free!(3)

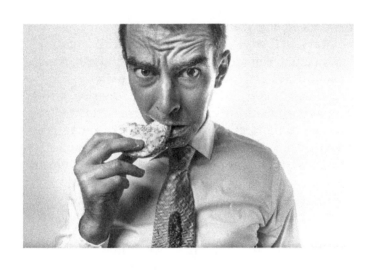

STEP 4: FOOD

You may have been tempted to skip the mind steps and go right towards the food step. If that's true, you made a bad decision. The mind is the first place where transformation begins. Once you get your head in the game, it becomes easier to get the food and exercise steps under control.

I am not here to introduce you to one specific diet. I am not here to promise you a method of eating that will change your life. I am here to give you some pointers on foods that will assist you with your health and weight loss. Making wise food choices is a major step to get down in order to see the transformation truly begin. I believe America has a problem when it comes to food. We are addicted. We love our extra-large portions. We love to eat until we are stuffed. We want our money's worth of food if we go out to a restaurant. We use food as entertainment. I believe food has become something that it was never intended to be. Instead of viewing food as nourishment, food has become an addiction and an idol. We aren't eating to live; we are living to eat.

The food step in my The ONE STEP Method is a simple one. Go natural and use moderation. Man-made foods should not be your main choices. I am going to give you 10 commandments to help you take this step.

The 10 Food Commandments
Commandment #1 Eat Natural/Organic

Natural is better than processed. I believe we all can agree that man-made foods are not as good for you as natural whole foods. What's even better? Natural whole organic foods. These foods can get expensive, so if you can afford organic, go for it. Buying local helps ensure that you are truly getting organic.

Most processed foods tend to have added salt and sugars. They may also be saturated with trans fats, which are not good for your body. Do your body a favor and begin eating natural foods. Natural foods consist of fruits, vegetables, healthy grains, eggs, meats, dairy, nuts, etc. Most grocery stores place their natural foods on their outer perimeter, while processed foods are the middle of the store. You should also beware of the word "natural". Some food companies like to use the word "natural" as a marketing strategy. Sugars can be natural, but they should be consumed in moderation. The same goes for fats. Do your homework and educate yourself on what is truly natural and what isn't.

Commandment #2 Protein is a must.
You should always eat protein at every meal. It's something that you should get used to doing. Make it a normal part of your meals. Protein sources are not hard to come by. Animal products are full of proteins. Animal proteins are a complete source of protein and filled with essential amino acids for optimal metabolism function, and muscle building. There are some vegan options, as well. Some plant proteins include beans, legumes, and soy. However, soy is usually heavily genetically modified; make sure you look for Non-GMO soy. Plant protein sources lack some amino acids that your body needs. Aim to get about 15-20 grams of protein per meal.

Commandment #3: Eat Your Vegetables.
Just saying the word "vegetables" can make you remember what Mom said. She always wanted you to eat your vegetables at the dinner table. Mom was

onto something. Did you know that vegetables are full of vital nutrients for your body? Studies have even shown that regular vegetable consumption has the potential to significantly decrease your risk of heart disease and cancer. Vegetables are a blessing from the Lord. We should aim to eat a variety of vegetables. A good rule of thumb is to aim to eat the rainbow. Dark leafy greens, and purple, red, orange, and yellow vegetables all have nutrients that will aid your body in getting healthier and fighting hunger. Vegetables can be eaten in a variety of ways. I prefer to eat fresh or frozen. Often times, canned vegetables are filled with sodium and BPA from the can lining. Not a vegetable person? Try them in a smoothie. Most of the time, you can't even tell that there's a serving of baby spinach in that vanilla peanut butter smoothie. Try to have a vegetable at every meal. Avoid emphasizing starchy vegetables, such as corn and potatoes. Eat those in moderation.

Commandment #4: Eat 5-6 meals per day (Portion control).

When you read that I encourage people to eat 5-6 meals per day, you may think I am nuts. How can you lose weight eating so frequently? It's simple. You space out your meals throughout the day to keep you satisfied, and to get your metabolism functioning at an optimal level. Try to eat a breakfast upon waking, a snack after a workout, a lunch, a light snack in the day, and dinner filled with protein and vegetables. An example of my menu looks like this:

Meal 1: 2 organic free range eggs with 2 egg whites, 1 serving of cheese and peppers and onions.

Meal 2: Protein bar (2 grams of sugar or less, and minimally processed.)

Meal 3: 1 serving of low-fat cottage cheese + 4oz grass-fed hamburger with onion, tomato, lettuce, mustard, and mayonnaise on a whole wheat pita pocket.

Meal 4: 1 cup of strawberries, 1-2 servings of celery, 1 serving of peanut butter

Meal 5: Large salad filled with baby spinach, romaine lettuce, iceberg lettuce, onions, peppers, fresh mushrooms, tomatoes, shredded cheese, bacon bits, 1 tablespoon of sunflower seeds, 1 can of tuna, oil and balsamic vinegar, salt and pepper, garlic and lemon zest. As you can see, you can get creative with spices. If you cannot stomach oil and vinegar, find a dressing with 2 grams of sugar or under and use just one serving. The less processed the better.

Meal 6: (Only if I am hungry) 3 hard-boiled egg whites

The sky's the limit with your foods. Just eat normal sized portions. Eat until you're satisfied. If you overeat, don't beat yourself up. Make sure you eat normal the rest of the day. Go for an extra walk to offset the calories consumed. Don't look at it as a punishment. Consider that you are blessing your body by helping it burn the extra fuel.

Side note: Begin to track your food. You'll begin to see how much you are eating, and how healthy your eating has become. You'll get to see what you eat too much of, or what you eat too little of. Track your food intake even if you overeat. It will give you a visual of what you are eating. Tracking food is a way to see your progress and your shortcomings. It allows you to observe yourself so you can rehabilitate your method of eating.

Commandment #5: Water is good.
I cannot stress enough how important water is for you. Please consume water as your first choice of a beverage. I make sure when I go out to eat to always ask for water. I rarely order anything else. Adding lemon to your water will make the flavor refreshing and it will even add some nutrients to your water. Try experimenting with water. Start by pouring water into a pitcher and slicing your favorite fruits to add to the water. Allow the fruits to soak in the water overnight, and the next morning you will have tasty fruit infused water. Water will do wonders for your health. It helps your skin, it can thin your blood, and it helps you feel satisfied. Sometimes, all we need is a glass of water to help the hunger pangs to pass.

Commandment #6: Avoid artificial sweeteners.
　　This goes along with our previous commandment. Many people believe wholeheartedly that diet soda or zero calorie drinks are okay to drink and guzzle down. Not so! Artificial sweeteners should be kept to a minimum. Studies have suggested that consumption of artificial sweeteners can lead to health problems and weight gain. Learn to develop your taste buds to prefer natural before unnatural flavors. Once your tastes become adapted to the natural, you won't even appreciate the taste of artificial flavors any longer. I've experienced this. I use to love the taste of regular soda. I stopped

drinking sodas and replaced them with water and coffee. I try regular soda today, and I can't handle the disgustingly sweet taste. You can get to that point, too. If you are drinking diet drinks and you can't imagine quitting, take a step back from consuming them by reducing how many you consume per day. Ween your way off of the diet drinks and onto natural alternatives. They will become your new go-to.

Commandment #7: Carbohydrates are cool.
When I say carbohydrates, you may think that they aren't good for you. Carbohydrates have also been given a bad rap lately. Carbohydrates can be broken down into simple carbs, and complex carbs. Simple carbs include sugars, honey, fruit, fruit juice, etc. Complex carbs are foods such as rice, wholegrains, whole wheat breads, etc. Fibers include most vegetables, greens, cauliflower, etc.

The majority of your carbs should come from vegetables. They are filled with fiber to keep you full and to regulate digestion. You want to eat moderate amounts of complex carbs, such as grains. Keep them to one serving, for best results. I recommend eating your carbs in the morning to early afternoon. This may help you avoid the mid-afternoon crash. Keep simple carbs to a minimum for the best weight loss transformation. They should be used as treats.

I want us to understand that carbs are not the enemy. They are necessary to give us energy. Consume them to get that energy. They are great to eat before a workout, and even after a good workout. Paired with some protein, they can help repair your muscles after a workout.

Commandment #8: Mix it up.

Try to mix your foods. Don't stick to the same old foods for the rest of your life. It will get boring, and it can lead you to stay away from your new healthy lifestyle. I recommend adding a new food or two every month. If you run out of food ideas, try a new spice. There are countless recipes that you can try to keep your taste buds content with a natural way of eating. Experiment! You'll appreciate variety. It's easy to get bored of the same old tastes. Search Pinterest or Google for healthy natural food ideas. Try soups. Try bakes. Try something in its natural state. You are only limited by your imagination when it comes to food choices. By mixing it up, you may find you now like foods that you didn't like before. Congratulations! You've just experienced transformation in your taste buds!

Commandment #9: Cheat

Did I say that right? Are we really allowed to do this? Yes! I recommend it. I recommend doing this after you get to a point where you are certain that your tastes have changed. Cheating can be done in multiple ways. You can have something that you know you shouldn't once per week or once per month. Or, you can follow the 90/10 rule. Eat natural and healthy food about 90 percent of the time, and have something not so natural 10 percent of the time. With the ONE STEP Method, we don't want to tell you what you can and cannot eat. We simply offer solutions that have the potential to give you the best results in the quickest amount of time. You may not be ready to give up all unnatural foods. I want to be the first to tell you that it's okay to be in that place.

Begin replacing them slowly. Try replacing an unnatural food with a natural food once or twice per week. You will notice by the end of a few months, you have made some big strides to success. We have to do this one step at a time. This isn't a comparison game. This is you becoming the best version of yourself. Sometimes it takes more than a day, a week, a month, or even a year to make that happen.

Commandment 10: Consider your Eating Methods

Your body burns calories differently depending on the type of food you consume. When you eat complex carbs and proteins, your metabolism becomes charged up and ready to burn glucose. Try to stay around 40 grams or less when you consume carbs, because they cause a spike in blood sugar. Also, it's best to keep your fat grams to a minimum when you consume carbohydrate/protein meals. I don't recommend these meals often. Once or twice per day is best, in my opinion.

Another type of eating method is eating fat and protein. An example of this type of meal would be having beef with cheese and mayo on a low carb wrap or bun. When you eat a higher fat meal along with protein, try not to eat complex carbohydrates with this meal. Get your carbohydrates from vegetables, such as greens. By eating in such a way, your body will burn fat differently by using different fuels from your foods. Eating like this, provides some variety so you don't feel like you're restricting yourself. This helps your body metabolize fats and carbs in a way that maximizes fat loss.

Another method would be to eat slowly. Often times we like to eat as quickly as possible. Take a time out and begin being conscious about how fast you are eating. Take smaller bites. Try to stop eating as if it's the first meal you've eaten in a year. By eating slower, you'll learn to enjoy food in a different way. This is another part of transformation.

Bonus Commandments:
Eat Fiber (Elaborating on Commandment #7):
It's insane how the modern American diet does not include enough fiber. It is recommended that men get 30-38 grams of fiber per day, and women should get 25 grams of fiber daily. Women who are 51 and older should consume roughly 21 grams of fiber day. Fiber not only helps you regulate bowel-movements, but it also keeps your cholesterol numbers in check, helps you break down your foods, cleans your intestines, decreases risk of cancer, and more. Vegetables, fruits, beans, and healthy grains contain fiber. Try to add fiber to your daily menu. Your body will thank you.

Food over supplements:
Some supplements can be helpful for success. Supplements can deliver some vital nutrients to your body, however, I do believe you should get your main nutrients from food. Supplements should come after. A rule that I live by is food first, supplements second.

Eat Only Until Content:
Many people want to eat until they are stuffed. This is a bad idea if you want to lose weight. You should eat until you are satisfied. When you consume way too many calories in one sitting, it makes you tired, uncomfortable, and sluggish. Eat until content, and stay energized and comfortable. Try to eat slowly. Put your fork/spoon down after every bite. Chew slowly, and sip some water as you eat. Water consumption helps you digest your foods better, and may help you get satisfied from that meal a little quicker. Aim for a feeling of contentment following a meal. Don't live to eat, eat to live.

Surrender:
America has a food addiction problem. We are addicted to the flavors and the taste. We are addicted the sentimental value of certain foods. If you are a Christian who struggles with food addiction, I wholeheartedly believe this is an area that you haven't fully surrendered over to Jesus. This may be a truth that you have a hard time admitting, but it's worth considering. If you want to experience freedom from food addiction, admit that you have a problem, then ask God to take control of this area of your life and direct your efforts to change. Pray and seek the Lord on this matter. Ask others for sound counsel. When you surrender the power to change your addiction over to God, you are no longer a slave to it. You tell it what to do, instead of it telling you what to do.

Now that you know the 10 Commands of the ONE STEP Method when it comes to food, apply them. Begin cleaning up your eating and watching the weight melt right off. Take small steps with these commandments, focusing on one at a time so you won't feel overwhelmed. After you master one, move on to the next. This will help you stay consistent and moving forward. Now, take a few minutes to record your reactions to the commandments and plan your next step.

What commandments will you work on first? Why?

What commandments will be the hardest to work on? Why?

What commandments do you want to add to the 10?

I'd like to introduce to you some of my top 10 lists for BREAKFAST/LUNCH/DINNER/SNACKS. How you combine your foods truly matters. You should eat strategically so you can maximize your weight loss. Here's a list of my top five foods in each category.

Note: All are individual servings.

Breakfast

Meal 1: One Step Omelet
2 Free-range chicken eggs , 2 egg whites – Scrambled
Add in: 1 serving of pepper jack cheese or Colby jack cheese
Add in: 1 serving of green peppers, jalapeños, onions
Add in: a pinch of salt and ground pepper
Protein: 24 grams

Meal 2: Pancakes
½ cup of 100% oats
1 tablespoon of ground flax
½ cup of low-fat cottage cheese
½ cup of egg whites
2 tablespoons of Truvia sweetener
Sprinkle of nutmeg
Sprinkle of cinnamon
1 drop of vanilla extract
Blend together and scoop onto pan to cook like a pancake.
Protein: 21 grams

Meal 3: French Toast
2 free-range chicken eggs
¼ cup of almond milk (unsweetened)
1 t spoon of vanilla extract
1 t spoon of nutmeg
45 calorie slice bread or Ezekiel bread
Mix batter together. Coat bread with batter and fry over butter.
Protein: 19 grams

Meal 4: Justin's Smoothie That Shapes Your Booty!
Almond milk Unsweetened (8-12 ounces)
½ cup of blackberries
½ cup of blueberries
½ cup of raspberries
1 cup of baby spinach
1 cup of vanilla or strawberry fat free Greek yogurt
Blend together and serve chilled.
Protein: 20 grams

Meal 5: Amazing Chocolate Peanut Butter Protein Pudding!
Almond milk unsweetened (8 ounces)
Low sugar chocolate whey protein powder (1 ¼ serving)
1 tablespoon of chocolate cocoa powder
1 teaspoon of vanilla extract
1 tablespoon of PB2
Directions: Shake all ingredients together for 1-2 minutes until it gets thick. Add more protein powder for a thicker texture.
Protein: 25 grams

Lunch

Meal 1: Taco Salad
Any type of salad mix (As much as you'd like)
Chopped Onion, Chopped Green pepper, Chopped tomato
1 serving of black beans
1 serving of ground beef (preferably grass fed)
Taco chips (healthy version would be baking a low-carb wrap until crispy and breaking up into salad)
No sugar added salsa
1 serving of sour cream
Protein: 23 grams

Meal 2: Ramen Noodles
1 Serving of Konjac Noodles
1.5 Cups of chicken broth
1 serving of cooked chicken breast (finely chopped)
Season with garlic powder, onion powder, parsley flakes.
Protein: 24 grams

Meal 3: Super Salad
Any type of salad mix (As much as you'd like)
Chopped onion, chopped red pepper, chopped yellow pepper, chopped carrots, chopped tomatoes, chopped walnuts, a small serving of sunflower seeds and almond pieces
Extra Virgin Olive Oil and Balsamic Vinaigrette Dressing (mixed with parmesan cheese, salt, pepper, and garlic)
Protein: 15 grams

Meal 4: Fiber-licious Lunch
Black beans, Konjac Noodles, Broccoli, Cauliflower, Minced Garlic, Butter to flavor, and Parmesan cheese to flavor. Pan fry in butter.
Protein: 15 grams of protein

Meal 5: Tuna Salad Roll-up
1 can or package of tuna (drained)
1-1.5 serving of organic mayo
Chopped celery, onion, carrots, cucumbers
Mix together and season to taste.
Place mix onto large Romaine lettuce leaves.
Protein: 18 grams

Dinner

Meal 1: Keep Me Full Salad
Salad greens (as much as you'd like.)
Chopped celery, tomatoes, onion, peppers, mushrooms
1-3 slices of natural bacon (chopped)
1 serving of ground chicken (seasoned to taste)
1 serving of shredded cheese
1 serving of Ranch dressing
Protein: 30 grams

Meal 2: Stir fry
Mixed vegetables (avoid too much corn)
Onions, Mushrooms, Peppers Jalapeño's, (chopped)
1 serving of black beans
1 serving of peanuts (no shell)
4oz chicken breast
Protein: 35 grams

Meal 3: Bacon-wrapped Steak Burger
4 oz. of grass fed beef steak cut(lean)
3 pieces of natural bacon (wrap around the beef)
1 slice of pepper jack or Colby jack cheese or Bleu cheese crumbles
Tomato slices, Banana pepper slices, Onion, Romaine lettuce.
1 serving of Joseph's Lavash Bread
Protein: 30 grams

Meal 4: Stuffed Peppers
4 ounces ground beef or chicken (grass fed or free range)
Chopped veggies into the ground meat
Add parmesan cheese into ground meat.
Slice pepper in half, fill raw pepper with meat.
Cover ground meat with natural (no-sugar added) tomato sauce.
Bake until pepper is soft.
Protein: 24 grams

Meal 5: One Step Pizza Mania
1 piece of lavash bread
Tomato sauce (no added sugar)
Add mozzarella cheese
Add veggies (as much as you'd like)
Add pepperoni, natural sausage, chicken (ground or breast)
Bake until desired
Protein: 20 grams

Snack foods:
Almonds (Natural is best, but salt and vinegar flavor are my favorite)
Sardines (in water, add your own mustard or hot sauce.)
Pork rinds (Plain – Dip in salsa or a serving of sour cream)
Fruit Salad Yogurt (Add berries to fat free Greek yogurt)
Cheese and berries (Cheese stick and a cup of your favorite berries)
Protein shakes (try to find protein shakes with 2 grams of sugar and under)
Protein bar (try to find a protein bar that has less sugar)

Again, ONE STEP does not give you a specific diet plan to follow. It helps you clean up your diet in small steps. ONE STEP is simple. Once you master one step, you'll want to master another. This makes it doable and not overwhelming.

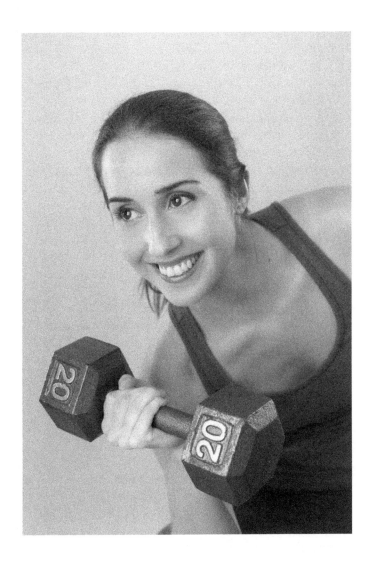

STEP 5: EXERCISE

This step is a very important part of the transformation process. Without exercise, you'll miss out on benefits of a healthier heart, higher metabolism, strength increase, a toned body, fat loss, etc. Exercise is a great partner to accompany your better food choices. Your choice to eat healthy, along with exercising to burn calories, will bring you beneficial maximum results.

The ONE STEP Method of exercise is going to help you see that exercise doesn't have to be a part of your day that you dread. You can actually enjoy an exercise session. How do you get to this level? Simple. You begin exercising in a way that fits your schedule and your fitness level. You'll begin to see progress and results, and you'll want to stick with exercising because it brings you the results.

Let me share a little about my exercise background. At 799lbs, my fitness level was obviously not at a point where I could use cardio machines, walk a mile, or even strength train. I was at a place where just standing up and sitting back down was a challenge for me. I would stand up, and sit back down three to six times. This was a struggle for me, but as I continued doing this particular exercise, I began getting stronger. I was able to do more, and eventually I felt more strength in my legs. The next exercise I mastered was walking. I was given a goal by my physical therapist to walk a mile as quickly as I could. It took me over 30 days to complete my first mile in steps. Eventually, I began getting my mile done quicker the next time around. I am now able to run and even walk up a steep incline. If I wouldn't have challenged myself, I wouldn't be where I am today. It hurt, yes. It caused me pain and sweat, yes. But I am glad that I persevered and continued on the road to recovery by exercising.

I recommend starting at the fitness level that you are at right now. I wouldn't recommend going to the gym and jogging a mile if you haven't been off the coach for a normal leisure walk in a while. If you are significantly overweight or have health problems, I recommend consulting with a physician before even starting a program. Once you get a doctor's permission, here is where you start.

Test yourself. Begin by just taking a leisure walk. Immediately after completing that walk, rate how you feel. Use the exertion scale, 1 to 10; 1 being a level where it was super easy, and you're not winded at all, 10 being a level where you just felt like you went all out and have nothing left. Once you can pin point a number where you are at, you'll want to begin seeking out an exercise program that is customized to you. We offer a Monthly Coaching Transformation Program to help with this on an individual level. You can visit www.onestepnation.com for more information on this program.

Let me share a few sample workouts for beginners.

Workout week sample.

Day 1: 5-10 minute walk or walk in place. (exertion scale of 5-6)
Stand up and sit down at your chair 3 sets of 12 reps. (Rest until you can go again.)

Day 2: 5-10 minute walk or walk in place (exertion scale of 5-6)
Wall pushups 3 sets of 12.

Day 3: Rest

Day 4: 5-10 minute walk or walk in place (exertion scale of 5-6)
Stand up and sit down at your chair 3 sets of 12 reps. (Rest until you can go again.)

Day 5: 5-10 minute walk or walk in place (exertion scale of 5-6)
Wall pushups 3 sets of 12.

Day 6: Rest

Day 7: 5-10 minute walk or walk in place (exertion scale of 5-6)
Front leg kicks 3 sets of 12 (each leg)
Shoulder press 3 sets of 12 (use weighted objects.)

The next week, you would add time to your walking minutes, or you could add a faster pace at intervals during your walk. For instance, you may want to aim for at least a minute of walking at an exertion level of 8-9 instead of 5-6. This will challenge your body in a new way.

    Adding small amounts of exercise and increasing gradually in time and intensity makes exercise doable for everyone. It does not have to be a task that makes you suffer. It can be a task that encourages you when you see results. Working out is now a part of my life that I never want to give up. I enjoy it because it's my time to spend reading my Bible, and also getting my body healthier. I want to see better quality of life, and longevity. I also understand that exercising should never get so easy that I am no longer challenged. Once something becomes too easy for you, it's time to step it up and add a challenge. Always challenge your body. Without a challenge, there is no transformation.

Some good beginner exercises to pick from are the following.

Bike pedaling (get a stationary pedal device to pedal while watching TV.
Walking
Wall push-ups
Wall sits
Water exercises
Stationary bike
Stand up and sit down
Step ups
Hula Hoop balancing on your arms
Overhead triceps extension with weight
Bicep curls
Resistance band training
Front kicks
Back kicks
Small squats
Step in, Step out
Walk in place
Half sit ups (lay on your bed, legs on the floor. (Push your body up in sit up position)
Calf raises
Punches/jabs
Standing core twist
Shoulder press
Triceps kickback
Hammer bicep curl

Reverse bicep curl
Exercise ball balancing
Sit-ups on exercise ball
Exercise ball bouncing
Sitting leg lifts
Squat to calf raise

Those are just a few exercises to pick from to start. Try them all out. Google or YouTube form and how to best do the exercise. By completing the exercises mentioned, you will be on your way to becoming a stronger, healthier you.

Next, you'll need to understand that there are different types of exercise. Cardiovascular exercise is one type. Strength training is another. High Intensity Interval Training (HIIT) is another method. All three offer benefits in their own unique way.

Examples of cardiovascular exercise:
Walking
Running
Jogging
Jumping
Jumping Jacks
Basketball
Stair climber
Elliptical
Jogging in place
Aerobics

Examples of strength training
Bench press
Leg press
Squats
Dead lifts
Shoulder press
Lateral shoulder raise
Triceps extension
Bicep curl

An example of HIIT (High Intensity Interval Training):
Pick four different exercises (called a circuit) and perform one after another at an intensity that is challenging. Rest only when you need to. This type of activity burns more calories and builds muscle in a shorter amount of time.

Circuit Examples
Jumping Jacks
Push-ups
Squats
Plank
Repeat 4 times, 12-15 reps each session

Wall Sit
Squats
Push-ups
Burpees/Full body extension
Repeat 4 times, 12-15 reps each session

Ways to get some interval training while doing cardiovascular exercise.
Plan a 30-minute walk.
5 minute warm up (exertion level of 3-4)

2 minute (exertion level of 5-6)
1 minute (exertion level of 8-9)
Repeat steps 2 and 3 seven times.
5-6 minute cool down walk (exertion level of 1-2)

     This type of exercise can be done outside or on a cardio machine. It's encouraged to always challenge yourself to get to the next level during your transformation. If something gets easier, increase the amount of time or the intensity. Add something that will challenge you to get your heart rate up and that will build muscle. Keep in mind that exercise is your friend. Treat it like it's a friend who wants to give you a better quality of life. Take a few minutes right now to reflect on your thoughts about exercise.

What are some exercises that you can start with right now?

What fitness level are you?

Where do you want to see yourself in 90 days when it comes to fitness? Be realistic.

Additional notes.

If you don't know where to start, just move! Do something, no matter how little of an effort you put into it. Most of the time at the beginning, you'll have to choose to work out, because it won't come naturally to just want to do it. Walk up and down the street. Take the steps. Park further away. Your body was created to move. The more active you decide to become, the stronger you will get.

Many question how to fit in exercise if they are working full time. There are plenty of ways to exercise when you are at work all day. You can still exercise, so please stop making excuses. Excuses will not give you success. You will just stay in the same condition until you decide to do something about it. Don't let your schedule ruin your journey to transformation.

Work week workouts:
Stand up and walk every hour – at least 2 minutes.
Stand up and sit down at your desk chair – 12-15 times per hour.
Use a standing desk.
Walk on your lunch break instead of sitting (take a quick lunch)
Stair climbing (you can use the stairs for a workout – aim for 5-20 minutes)
Desk pushups
Squats

The sky's the limit. You are your only limiter. You can see results by just applying a few of the exercises above. I started at 799 lbs. I could have made every excuse in the world. I didn't though, I just kept going. I didn't want to be 799 lbs. anymore. Are you tired of being in the condition that you are in? It's time to get moving. No more excuses. Only forward steps. What are you waiting for? Move it!

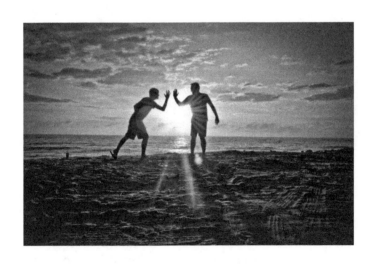

STEP 6: ACCOUNTABILITY/SUPPORT GROUP

This step was a huge contributor to my success. Once you start your journey, you'll want to develop a type of support group. ONE STEP offers an online community with our coaching program to give you that accountability. When a person holds you accountable, it will help you stay on track.

Here are five benefits of an accountability partner.

1. Encouragement: Everyone needs encouragement here and there. I had an accountability partner who would encourage me nearly every single day. I would inform her what my wins were, or what my positive steps were, and she would encourage me to keep going. She would celebrate with me over the phone. She would pray for me, and would always speak positively about me, knowing my intentions were to lose weight and to become healthier. Encouragement can help us go the extra mile. If you are the person holding someone accountable, remember, words can build someone up or tear someone down. Our heart should always be ready to build someone up. When someone feels supported, they will feel happy and ready to tackle any obstacle that is in front of them.

2. Inspiration: Ask your accountability partner to inspire you by sending you some inspirational quotes, Bible verse, prayers, images, etc. Tell them what inspires you, and ask them if they would help you by sending inspiring texts, e-mails, and phone calls, so you can continue to move forward on your ONE STEP journey.

3. Support: Knowing that the person who is holding you accountable supports you, it gives you the feeling that someone is for you. If you know someone is for you, you'll win the fight against your destructive desires. We are stronger together.

4. Accountability: Someone to hold you accountable doesn't sound all that fun. But it will help you stay on track. It's easy to quit and give up without someone checking in on you. A lot of people don't like having others in their business. Find someone you trust enough to hold you accountable. Give them three questions to ask you every single day. For example, they might ask you, "Did you get your activity in today? Did you only eat foods that you're allowed to eat on your plan today? How's your mindset? Is your head in the game? What can I do to help? What can I be praying about for you? Did you speak positive about yourself today?" Do not take offense at what they ask or say. Remember they are helping you see transformation.

5. Challenge: Ask your accountability partner to give you a weekly challenge. Maybe it includes exercising more or switching up your routine. Maybe it means trying a new food, or eating less. Have them issue you a challenge so you can rise up and experience a push towards your transformation goal. Remember, without challenge, there is no growth.

Support groups are also a big part of success. I had a group of people around me who would support me on my journey. I would walk around Walmart several times per week and I built relationships with the staff. They would always encourage me when I would see them. They supported my Walmart walking sessions. They would be cheering me when they saw me approaching. I also had a church family who supported me on my journey. They helped me by praying for me, sending me inspirational notes, holding me accountable, and more.

You should establish a support group so you also can reach your goals easier. There is just something about having a support group that makes you feel like you're not alone on your journey. Here are some ideas of support groups you could reach out to.

ONE STEP Monthly Coaching Transformation Program: You can join our coaching program to find support from myself and my partners. We support you every step of the way. ********

ONE STEP 9-Week Course: One Step offers a 9-week course with those who want basic information on how to see transformation in their mind, body and spirit. The course helps people establish a healthy relationship with their health.

Church: Church families are a great support. Having people who share your beliefs will help you feel supported. Find a church that loves God and loves people. Get involved and develop relationships with brothers and sisters.

Weight loss clubs: Gyms, clubs or workout classes are great ways to develop a support system. Mostly everyone who attends these have a common goal of improving health. Find some people you can connect with to help you develop a support group.

Online Support Groups: There are multiple online weight loss support groups. Try searching for them and joining them.

Family: Family can be a great support. Tell your family what you are trying to accomplish, and allow them to support you throughout your journey.

Don't run away from accountability. Don't skip this step and say you don't need it. If I were to have said this when I was on my journey to losing 600lbs, I wouldn't have done it. It took more than me to get through the obstacles that I faced. Try to be open minded. Drop the pride that is holding you back from getting a support group. Drop the insecurities that hold you back from developing friendships and accountability partners. We are all imperfect. Nobody has to remind us. Remember that we also will be building friendships and partnerships with those who also struggle. Don't let emotions or feelings hold you back from fulfilling this step. You will be glad that you chose to find an accountability partner, and a support group. Take a minute to brainstorm some ideas about your potential support system.

What are some support groups that you are aware of that you could get involved in?

1._____

2. _____

3. _____

Who are the people that you could ask to hold you accountable?

1._____

2. _____

3. _____

What are three questions I want them to ask me daily?

1._____

2._____

3. _____

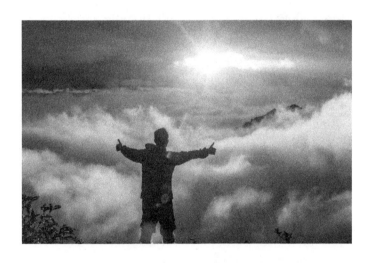

STEP 7: SPIRITUAL HEALTH

ONE STEP is not just about the body. It's also about the spirit. Without a healthy spirit, you won't have a healthy body. Healthy spirituality is an important factor in treating your body the way it deserves to be treated. It deserves to be treated as a gift.

I am a Christian. I believe in Jesus and I follow Him. I allow His approach to life to mold and shape me on my journey. I started following Jesus in August 2003. Every day, as I pray, read and spend time with Him, I begin to learn about Him in a deeper way. It's not just a religion to me, it's a relationship. The amazing thing is that I am nothing special. I am a person who is loved by my Heavenly Father. It's an unconditional love, because Lord knows that I don't deserve it. I want you to understand that I am not here to force my faith on you. However, I will mention it, as it is a part of my life. I'll also mention it because I believe once you recognize your worth and value, you'll have an easier time getting the rest of your life in order. Not just your health, but also your finances, relationships and so much more.

Spiritual health at its peak, gives us a trickle-down effect. Once you feel on top of the world spiritually, and you begin to feel really connected to God, you'll have a different outlook on life. It suddenly becomes apparent that the way we live, the methods we use, the way we treat our bodies – it all lines up with how God would want us to treat ourselves. It takes the eyes off of ourselves and onto Him and His design and intentions for our lives. Allow me to share what my faith did for me.

1. Purpose: I developed a feeling of purpose. I knew I existed for more than just breathing and taking up space. I trusted that God made me for a reason. I was here for a purpose and I was going to pursue God to find that purpose.

2. Value: When I gave my life over to Jesus, I began to notice that my value wasn't in my appearance. It wasn't in the clothes I wore, or the money I had in my pocket or bank account. My value was based on what He said about me. God loved me enough to die on a cross for my mistakes even when I was stubborn and selfish and rebellious. He restored me back to a perfect relationship with Him because Jesus took my mistakes that offended God, who told me not to make them. Jesus said I am worth dying for. I am very thankful that I have value and worth in Him.

3. Casting my cares on Him: I had extreme anxiety attacks that plagued me with the fear of death. I would be afraid to move, because I thought my heart was going to give out on me. I was in constant stress because of the anxiety disorder. I learned to give Jesus all of my worries. I knew if I was to live or die, I would be with Him. I threw myself on Him in order to no longer be enslaved to anxiety. He takes it away. This is not to say that I never struggle with it, however, I know who helps me calm my anxiety. He keeps me in perfect peace.(4)

4. I am a gift: God created me. I am His gift to show Him to a world who is searching for Him. Some people don't even realize that they are searching for acceptance and love. They search for it in food, money, sex, drugs, alcohol, fame and more. We are a gift to show the love of God to others.

5. A story: God made a story out of me. My heart is always focused on helping others know The One who continues making my story. It's not about me, nor will it ever be. All eyes on Him.

6. Confidence: I am not confident in my own power or strength. But I am confident in Him. When I am feeling weak and overwhelmed, it's God who is strong through me. Confidence comes from my value and worth in Him. I don't have to worry about what others think of me. I only have to be concerned about what my Heavenly Father thinks of me. He thinks the world of me, like He thinks the world of you.

7. Forgiveness/No More Guilt: I am forgiven for all of my mistakes. I have a God who is faithful and just to forgive me and clean me of my wrongs against Him. He throws my mistakes away so He remembers them no more. I am walking before Him confidently. Sometimes I am tempted to beat myself up for having allowed myself to get so big. But guess what? I have no more guilt. He took that away. (5)

8. A New Creation: I am a new creation. The old me died when I accepted Jesus. The new me lives in Him. I am SON of God. I live in my sonship. I have value and worth because of my sonship. I matter because I am son of God. (6)

9. Others matter: It's not about me. Other people matter. I need to treat them the way that I want to be treated. I am to put others before myself. That's why I am writing this book. That's why I talk to people online about their struggles. That's why I share my faith with others. I care about others physically and spiritually. I don't just help them to better health, I also help them out from suffering an eternity separated from God. He loves us too much to have us go to hell. God never sends anyone to hell. We condemn ourselves because we reject Him. He offers His arms open to us at all times. It's never too late to say, "yes" to Him.

10. Eternity: I know where I am going when I take my last breath. I love Him. I am connected to Him. I know where my eternal home will be. I am very thankful for my relationship with Him.

Maybe you never thought too much about faith. You may identify yourself as a seeker or a maybe someone who "never really cared". Either way, I just want you to consider seeking out your Creator. He said if you seek Him with all of your heart, it's then you will find Him.(7) That doesn't mean to just try Him out, like you do when tasting a new food, that means to seek Him with everything you are, like searching for a treasure. You won't be disappointed.

How to seek God
1. Say, "yes" to God. Enter into a relationship with Him. Ask Jesus to rescue you from yourself and to come into your life. Ask Him to save you and to help you grow in a relationship with Him. Make a decision to devote your life to Him. Call Him Lord (which means The One in charge).

2. Pray: Prayer means talking to God. Just talk to Him. Don't worry about developing an elaborate prayer language. He just wants you to talk to Him.

3. Read your Bible: Read His word. It's His instruction manual to you and me. Start with one of the books of the gospels in the New Testament, such as John. You may read it and have questions, and that is okay. Just don't give up if something stumps you. Just keep going and God will answer the questions that you have. He will answer through His word, through prayer, through people, through dreams or visions. He is a BIG God. Don't underestimate Him. Just because you read something in the Bible that you don't agree with, doesn't mean it didn't happen. Also, just because we read something that appears off to us about God, that doesn't mean it is. There's always a reason why God says the things He did in the Bible. There's always a reason as to why He did what He did. Study to find those answers. Remember, you'll find Him if you seek Him with all of your heart.

4. Get connected to other believers: I highly recommend finding a church to become involved with. No church is perfect, because you're dealing with imperfect people. But don't forget, you aren't perfect, either. Build friendships and grow with others in your spiritual understanding.

Spirituality was a big contributor to my story. As you can see, my life has been changed. I am no longer the same person. It took 14+ years to get where I am at with Jesus today. Following Him and becoming like Him is a process. It's not an overnight thing. We are constantly learning, constantly seeking, and constantly yearning to become like Him. This will be lifelong. Never get fed up or frustrated. You are worth it to Him. He wants to mold and shape you into the best version of yourself that you can be through Him. Don't wait another minute. Give your heart over to Him. He loves you and is waiting. If you don't know what to say, use the prayer below.

Prayer: Father God, I want to thank you for your love that you have offered to me. I admit that I am not deserving. I admit that I have failed to live up to your expectations. I admit that I am powerless without you. I need your help. I ask Jesus to come into my life. Change me. Help me to live for you and to devote myself to you. Forgive me of my wrongs and help me to live a life that is honoring to you. I accept you, Jesus, as the One in charge of my life. From this day forward, I will choose to live for you. Give me the ability to follow you and to be like you. I pray this in the name of Jesus. Amen.

Write out your own prayer to God:

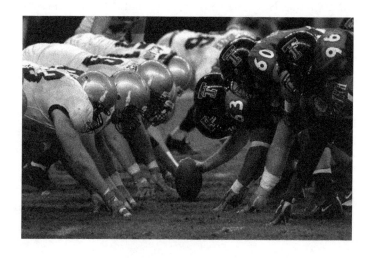

STEP 8: MIND/BODY/SPIRIT (OFFENSE AND DEFENSE)

It's easy to look at ourselves and immediately place all of our attention on our body. We often neglect the bigger issues that we struggle with. Often times what we see in the mirror is a result of what's going on in our mind and in our spirit. I explained earlier that the mind is an important factor for success. Having a healthy spirit is also very important, because it will help us see things in a different light. A healthy spirit helps us develop a healthy body. If one of the three is out of whack, we won't be functioning to our fullest potential.

We will need a healthy mind to help us be on our offensive game and defensive game when it comes to our thoughts. We will have negative thoughts that bombard our minds with trash that will make us feel hopeless or insecure. We will even begin to feel like giving up and taking steps backwards. Having a healthy mind will help us develop methods to fight off the attack.

<u>Healthy Thoughts to Maximize Your Success:</u>
1. Remind yourself that you matter: This will allow you to tell everything else such as food, or any other temptations to get off your back. You matter. Food addiction makes us treat ourselves as if we don't matter. You're worth more than a moment of food on your lips. We can have a powerful offense to attack the temptation with truth, telling our minds that we do matter, that we aren't hopeless and actually believing it. When we choose to believe it, it sets up a shield for defense, so more negative thoughts can't

come back and plague us into a negative state of mind.

2. Remind yourself that you are a work in progress: Progress doesn't happen overnight. It will be easy to think that it should. It could take weeks, months, or even years to see total transformation, even by applying all ONE STEP steps. Progress will require patience. You will need to develop a mindset of being patient with yourself. There is no magic formula that gives you results overnight. I wish that were the case. If it were true, I would have lost 600lbs more quickly than I did. It took me over 8 years to get to where I felt comfortable with my body. It's taken me 14 years to develop the continuing habits to remain healthy and fit. I don't set up unrealistic expectations. Progress happens one day at a time. Don't get impatient. Have patience with yourself.

3. It's On You
You need to develop a mindset that gives you ownership. When we fail, take ownership. When you succeed, recognize that you succeeded. Fact is, nobody will twist your arm to change. You have to make up your mind to do it. You will have to develop a frame of mind, knowing that nobody is going to force you to stop eating so much, or to exercise. You'll need to own it. You have to make the decisions to think the thoughts and act on the thoughts to help you experience success and full transformation. Thinking about blaming others for your lack of success will not help you. Fast food places didn't make you gain weight. Lacking a treadmill didn't make you gain weight. We all got ourselves into our own mess; we have to get ourselves out. Recognize

that and get that into your mind. It will help you take ownership of you and your actions. Here's a short recap of ONE STEP:

<u>Healthy Actions to Maximize Your Success:</u>
1. Eat Healthy: This is the obvious one. What you put into your mouth will either add to your current overweight condition, or it will help you escape your current weigh problem. A candy bar is going to add to your current condition. A healthy source of protein or a vegetable will set you up to get past your current condition. Choose healthier foods over unhealthy foods. Unhealthy foods equal an unhealthy body. Healthy foods equal a healthy body.

2. Get Moving: It's simple. The more you move, the better off you will be. Get active. Walk more. Get up and change the TV without the remote. Walk to work. Challenge yourself and do something that will get your heart beating faster. Moving doesn't have to be chore. Moving can become a normal part of your life. It doesn't have to be something you dread. It can eventually become something you look forward to.

3. Plan your meals/Plan your exercise: When we don't plan, we are basically planning to fail. Success requires planning your foods and your exercise sessions in order to maximize results. Without planning you may lose motivation. Without planning you may decide to get lazy. Write out your menu for the week. Write out your workouts for the week. Follow them and treat them like appointments that you can't miss. You'll see greater results by sticking to your plan.

4. Surround yourself with like-minded people: When you surround yourself with like-minded people, you'll surround yourself with good company. If you surround yourself with people who don't care about what they eat, you'll likely fall with them. If you surround yourself with people who are careless about their health, you will most likely begin feeling the same way about your health. People become who they surround themselves with. Healthy minded people surround themselves with other healthy minded people.

5. Accountability: If you lack accountability, you'll set yourself up for failure. Have you ever tried holding yourself accountable? It doesn't work very well. Find 1 or 2 people that you trust. Inform them what you are trying to do, and give them three questions to ask you regularly. If you don't hear from them, make sure you inform them how your day went. Answer the questions that you gave them. Don't put everything on the people holding you accountable. Put it in your hands.

<u>Healthy Spirituality to Maximize Your Success:</u>
1. Remember your value and worth: Remember that you have value and worth. Your Creator said so. He loves you and thinks the world of you. Operate out of that belief.

2. You are a son/daughter of the King: You are a son or daughter of God. Your Dad can help you through anything. Dad's want what's best for their children. Live to make your Dad proud.

3. Operate out of conviction and not emotions/feelings: This is hard for many people. If we feel overwhelmed, stressed, angry, sad, depressed, we will want to give into our temptations. Be led by your convictions over your emotions. Choose to operate out of what you believe is right and wrong. Don't allow emotions to rule. Emotions are gifts from God, but they should never lead us into making rash decisions.

4. Pray/Memorize Scripture: God has placed us in this world to live for Him. We should have constant communication with Him. We should write about Him by journaling. We should sing songs to Him as a form of worship. We should memorize His word and hide in our hearts, so we won't sin. We should meditate on His word day and night. He gave it to us to help us connect with Him and to learn His will for our lives. Memorize verses to help you make better decisions that please God before yourself and your desires. Write down prayers so you can read them and pray them from your heart. Journal what God is doing in your life. What is He asking? What has He been doing? What have you been learning? Get your focus off of fleshly desires and onto Him. It will change the game for you!

Applying these healthy principles in your mind, body and spirit, will help you stay focused on your journey to transformation. It's worth getting these three areas in order so that you won't be powerless against addictions, temptations and bad habits. You can overcome! You are a victor! You are not a victim!

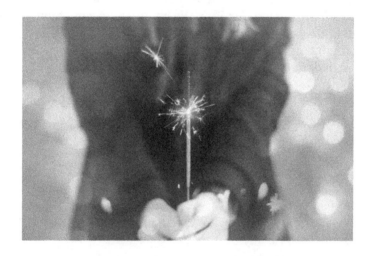

STEP 9: CELEBRATE

This is something we often fail to do. I love to celebrate! I love to see the success in my life. Did you lose a pound? Celebrate! Did you lose an inch? Celebrate! Did you memorize a scripture? Celebrate! Did you say, "no" to temptation? Celebrate! This is something we should do all of the time. By failing to celebrate, life can become a duty and a routine. On our transformation journey, life can become something we just do, like going through the motions. We are people, we need to be happy and be excited about our success. That helps us recognize results so we can create more and even greater results.

When I was losing pounds and inches fast, I had friends celebrate with me. They congratulated me for my hard work. They told me that they could tell that I was losing weight. They would high-five me, hug me, and treat me to movies, meals, buy me clothes, etc. It was all part of my support group that I had around me. They truly cared about me and supported me in the good times and bad times. Celebration was always a good time.

Now when it comes to celebrating, it is easy to think about food and food alone. It's easy to tell yourself that you did good, so you deserve a donut or a candy bar. But the fact is, we have to develop a new approach, especially if we want transformation to happen to the fullest. Why do we always go to food to celebrate? We know food is a commonality with most people. There is something about feasting that makes you happy. Food tickles the taste buds. Food releases feel good endorphins that make us happy. I believe food has become some sort of idol in the lives of people. It appears that it often becomes the center of attention at gatherings, or at celebrations. The truth is, it doesn't have to be. Here are some ways to celebrate without food.

Ways to Celebrate Without Food
1. Go to a movie: It's easy. A movie ticket costs just as much as fast food meal. Grab a movie ticket from your local theatre and go see a movie. You're not a person who likes to go alone? Grab a friend. If you have to have something in your hand? Grab a water or a coffee. Low calorie natural fruit drinks are also a good idea.

2. Start a collection: Start a collection of something that interests you. For some people it's football cards, for others it's coins. It all depends on what you are interested in. I have a TV series video collection that I like adding to. I am a sucker for 90's TV shows. I like to collect more of the 90's TV shows to watch instead of eating food that I don't need. I even invite my friends over to watch.

3. Buy new clothes: We will obviously need to buy new clothes when we begin to lose weight or build muscle. You can't afford new clothes? Check out your local thrift store where you can often find new clothes available to you for a great low price. Find an outfit that shows off your new confident personality.

4. Massage: It feels good. It can help you feel good in the same way that food makes you momentarily feel good. Massages can calm you down and help you get your mind off of food. Why not treat yourself to a stress-free moment instead of adding something to your body that will just add pounds and feed your addiction?

5. Intimacy with your spouse: Don't neglect this. Sex burns calories. Sex also feels good. So why not just be intimate with your spouse? You don't need food for a romantic evening. A glass of wine or 100% sparkling grape juice is relaxing to drink together. Enjoy each other the way God intended you to.

6. Share on social media: Share a before and after picture with your friends on social media. Let them know the win you are celebrating. They'll celebrate with you!

7. Vacation: Save your money that you'd normally spend on celebrating with food, and go on a vacation with your family. It'll be a relaxing time away from the stresses of life.

8. Start a weight loss club: Have you been changed by your success? Start a club to help other people. Starting a club will also hold you accountable and will keep you devoted to your new lifestyle. Meet once per week or once per month. Do this online or in person. So many people are looking for help. Be the help that they are looking for. Help yourself by helping them.

9. Tell your friends: Call a friend and let them know how awesome you are doing. Share with them how you overcame a bad habit or a bad thought. Share how you lost weight or inches. Telling someone helps you keep your head in the game.

Celebrating is fun! It doesn't have to involve food. We turn food into something it was never meant to be. It's time to kick that addiction to the curb. Hello celebration! Celebrate your wins in ways that will keep you in the mode of transformation! Take a few minutes now to think of alternate ways to celebrate.

What are some things to celebrate on your transformation journey?:

Why do you think food is a go-to celebration item?

What can you choose to do to celebrate your success?

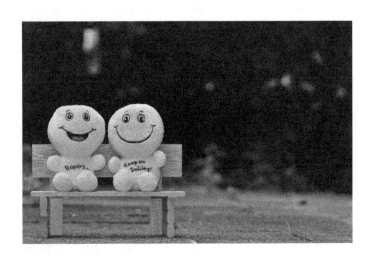

STEP 10: SHARE YOUR STORY

Here is the best part. Sharing your story of success keeps you in tune with your how far you've come. Any type of success is worth mentioning to others. There are many people who are in the situation you are in, and are looking for a way out. Why not be that beacon of hope to a person who doesn't know where to turn?

On my weight loss journey, I've had many opportunities to be part of some major platforms. I was in national and international magazines. I was on local news channels and national newspapers. I was given the opportunity to be on several TV shows, including *Inside Edition, The Today Show* and *The Doctors*. I was able to share my story with millions of people by just being open and by people seeing my success. I find no joy in living life in a way that's too private. I find that the healing is in the helping. There are people who were once in my shoes, and could use the help that I can offer them. Why would I withhold my story from them? I've had person after person inform me that my story touched their lives in a way that I couldn't imagine. God used my story to save someone from committing suicide. God used my story to help the morbidly obese find hope and to lose weight. If I didn't share this story, it would rob a lot of people of experiencing encouragement and freedom from their situation.

Why can't we be transparent? Why can't we drop our fake front and allow people to see the real us? Nobody is perfect. We've all struggled or are currently struggling with something. The question is, what will we do? Will we hide that we struggled or struggle? Or will we be open and honest and allow people to see our messiness? It's amazing that there is a message in the mess. What is the story in your history? There is hope, in your hopelessness. We don't need to be confined in a victim minded perspective. We are not victims. We are victors! Victors lead others to victory. When was the last time you shared your story with someone who was struggling with something you struggled with? Don't withhold hope from them any longer. Be the light in the darkness for them. Here are some ways to share your story.

1. Share your story on social media: Social media is an amazing place to start when it comes to sharing your story. There are millions of people on social media who are scrolling through their phones all day long. By sharing your story, it may catch someone's eye. This may be the moment they needed in order to get past their depression, hopelessness and situation because you chose to share your story with the world. By overlooking our pride, we allow people to see a formerly broken and messed up person just like them, and see hope! What if your story could help someone lose weight? What if it could help someone stop eating so much? What if they put that extra piece of pizza down because of your post? Think outside the box.

2. Discuss in person: Have you ever just shared your story with a stranger? I have, and it's fun. Sometimes they just act like it's a nice story, others will be shocked, and still others will inform me that that's exactly what they needed to hear. Our story can brighten up a day, transform a life and even help a person find hope in a hopeless situation. I've talked to morbidly obese people in person. It's always awkward at first to discuss myself with them, so I usually start the conversation out with asking their name. I'll take a few moments to hear from them and allow them to talk. I then share who I am and my story with them. They are usually pretty thankful that I did end up sharing with them.

Share with your church: Churches are usually willing to hear stories of people who have been changed. If you have a story that shows transformation and change, then it's time to share that. There are people in your church family who may be in the exact spot you are in. They are overweight and not sure where to turn for help. They are addicted to pornography, alcohol, drugs, etc., and they don't know where to turn to get help. You may be their answer to prayer. Share with them. It could change their lives and their eternity.

One Step Nation Facebook Page/Website: You can share your story with us at ONE STEP NATION on Facebook. You can simply go to www.facebook.com/onestepnation or even at our website at www.onestepnation.com. We'd love to hear from people who have been inspired and changed by the ONE STEP NATION to transformation. I'll get to see how well you are doing, and others will get to read about it, as well!

    I believe every story of success is worth sharing. Please remember that success is contagious. People want success, too. How do they get there? You may have that answer for them. Did Jesus change your heart? Share it. Did ONE STEP help you see transformation? Share it. Did you reach your goal weight? Share it. There's no time to keep silent. By helping others, you are helping yourself succeed and to stay in the moment of success. Take a few minutes to jot down your thoughts about how to share your experience.

What's your story?

FINAL WORDS

You may hear my story and be impressed. You may hear my story and not be impressed. The truth is, I am okay with either one of the responses. I don't do this for myself. I do this for those who may experience change because I shared my story with them. My hope is that you will read my story and end up being inspired in some way. I was a 14-year-old kid who struggled with anxiety attacks and food addiction. I allowed myself to stay inactive because of a fear of death. I coped with my anxiety and depression by eating an abundance of food. I ballooned up to 799lbs at the age of 16. I was a teenage boy who spiraled out of control and needed a different direction of life. Jesus rescued me from myself and I am forever thankful. It took me more than 8 years to shed 600 lbs. I was able to lose that weight and receive the blessing of free skin reduction surgery. Dr. Barry Debernardo, of New Jersey Plastic Surgery, has been a blessing to me with his services. I highly recommend him and his excellent staff to take care of any plastic surgery need.

I was able to share my story with media outlets nationally and internationally. This was not an accident, this was God's blessing on me. He allowed me to have a platform to show others hope; to point others to Him and to make Him famous by representing Him on all occasions. I am now 30 years old, and I am married to my beautiful wife. My wife and I are praying that God blesses us one day with children. I trust Him and believe He will. I Pastor a church in a small town. My church is called Open Arms Community Church. Our website is www.openarms.tv. I am constantly helping people by coaching them into better health. I created a coaching program designed to help you reach transformation, one step at a time. The program has been a success for many, and there's plenty of room for more success.

    My heart's desire is for people to get the help that they need. I am excited to see that my story has been seen and heard by millions of people. It's amazing to know that it has impacted people who I've talked to and many more who I haven't talked to. I am honored and humbled to be part of such an amazing story. I sit in awe of how good God is, and my wife and I are waiting in expectancy for the Lord to continue doing a good work with ONE STEP. Blessings, friends. Thanks for reading this book. I trust you will apply the principles that are at your fingertips. Please apply ONE STEP and begin your journey. Be patient with your progress. This now becomes a lifestyle. You can do it! I believe in you! Remember, it all starts with ONE STEP!
- Justin Willoughy
www.onestepnation.com

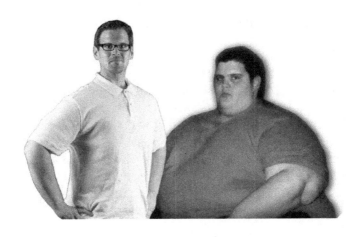

Bonus: How Justin Lost his Weight.

Here are my top 11 methods to weight-loss, One Step at a time.

1. Faith: It helped me refocus and it changed everything. I live for something bigger and better than addiction and food.

2. Moving: It wasn't easy, but I just began moving however I could. I would stand and sit. I would walk in place. I would walk a few steps and back to my bed. I would do any activity that I could to burn off the body fat that had me trapped in a prison.

3. Food: Portion size and moderation was the key to my success. I do no subscribe to any particular diet. I only subscribe to natural and whole foods. I am not a person who discourages carbs, fats, etc. I say eat them all in moderation. Veggies, fruits, proteins and healthy fats were key to my success. My diet didn't include white breads, cereals, rice, candy, chips and sweets. I had to eat those very sparingly to lose the weight that I lost. Sacrifice has to be made to see the best results.

4. Support: I was able to have people support me by praying for me, encouraging me and helping me through my tough times. I am forever thankful to my friend Melody Polluck who helped me through some of my hardest times. I am thankful for my parents and my brother for helping me to see that I was going to make it out of my rock bottom moment. I am thankful for the ambulance team who went to my house trailer to rescue me and take me Pittsburgh, PA Children's Hospital, so I could get the help needed. I am thankful for my mentors, Mike McAvoy, Larry Petry, Eric

Eliason, Mike Paterneti, Josh Hatcher, John Sheehan, Greg Newkirk, Scott Newton and many more. Those men poured out their time and knowledge into me. They have been very supportive throughout my life. They've helped tremendously when it comes to my success.

5. Accountability: I needed people to speak into my life. I needed people to hold me accountable. Without being held accountable, I'd continue to fall over and over again to food addiction. It took many phone calls, text messages and face to face moments, but I was able to find the accountability needed to overcome addiction. I encourage everyone to find someone who will hold them accountable.

6. Always Challenging Myself: I am never content with the easy way. I want something to challenge me. If the workouts become too easy, I have to challenge myself and make them harder. If the food in-take becomes too boring, I need to try new foods. If my muscle tone has decreased or has become stagnant, it's time to step it up a notch. Always push yourself to a new level. Challenge brings change.

7. Goal Setting: Set a weight loss goal for yourself. Set a diet goal for yourself. Set a spiritual goal for yourself. Setting goals will help you stay motivated. They will help you find success and stay on that road to success. Set a goal and stick to it.

8. Tracking Diet: I use a fitness tracker app to track my food intake. I watch what I eat. It helps me to know what I struggle with or if I am not eating enough veggies or protein.

9. Tracking Exercise: I use a fitness tracker app to track my exercise and activity. By tracking my activity for the day, I can see if I challenged myself or not. I can also see how far I've come by comparing my current workout to a workout that I did 30 days prior. If I haven't gotten better with something, I will push to get better.

10. Motivating Factors: I find three motivating factors that help me stay focused. By finding something that motivates me, I am more likely to stick to my transformation journey. My faith, my family, and my story are my motivators. I encourage everyone to find something that motivates them. Write them down and hang them up so they are constantly visible. Let them be a reminder of why you are trying to lose weight and get healthier.

Share your story: This is a must. Sharing helps you stay committed. Once someone knows your story, you don't want to go back. You want to continue to inspire and to help others. Now others look at you for help and to be the example. Sharing is a way to stay consistent on your journey.

JUSTIN'S RESOURCES FOR YOUR SUCCESS.

Justin Willoughby has lost 600lbs all naturally. It's his heart to help others experience weight loss, as well. It doesn't matter if you have 10 pounds to lose, or 1,000 pounds to lose. Justin offers his expertise on what you can do to help shed that unwanted weight, and to gain back confidence and happiness.

Here are a few tools Justin offers for success!

ONE STEP 9-Week Course: Available on www.onestepnation.com. Justin, along with his team of coaches, help individuals learn the basics of health and fitness. Justin takes individuals through a 9-week course of basic information to teach each person how to start their healthy journey. If you find yourself struggling with not knowing how to start, this One Step 9 -Week Course is for you. *****

Food Consumed Me: How I Overcame Food Addiction E-book: This book is to help those with a food addiction overcome that issue. Justin discusses his history with food. He gives readers a guideline to follow to overcome the addiction. The book is available on www.onestepnation.com or on www.justinwilloughby.com

Monday Mentality Book: This book helps those who cannot seem to shake the "I'll start Monday" mindset. Justin shares how he overcame the mindset, so he could start at the next meal, instead of starting in a few days. He teaches that just because you mess up once, doesn't mean the rest of the week is ruined. The book is available at www.onestepnation.com or www.justinwilloughby.com

ONE STEP Monthly Coaching Transformation Program: This program is designed to help individuals see success ONE STEP at a time. Justin and his team take you through the steps necessary to see success and transformation. Justin and his team help individuals to have victory on their health journey. The Monthly Coaching Transformation Program is unique, because it targets one area at a time. Justin and his team work closely with each person to ensure quality care and quality success. You can sign up at www.onestepnation.com or inquire for more information. *******

The THRIVE Experience: Justin Willoughby believes that supplements can be used as tools to help people reach their goals. He doesn't believe that supplements are the answer for success, but are looked at as enhancers along the journey. Justin offers a product that helps him get through his workouts, helps him shed unwanted weight, get past hunger spells, and that helps him have energy. You can see more about this product at www.onestepnation.com/thrive

If you have any questions regarding ONE STEP programs or E-books, please send email to onestepnation@gmail.com.

Notes:
1. Romans 12:2
2. Proverbs 23:7
3. John 8:32
4. Isaiah 26:3, Philippians 4:6,7
5. I John 1:9
6. 2 Corinthians 5:17
7. Deuteronomy 4:29